SURGERY - PROCEDURES, COMPLICATIONS, AND RESULTS

MINIMALLY INVASIVE SURGERY FOR PITUITARY ADENOMA

SURGERY - PROCEDURES, COMPLICATIONS, AND RESULTS

Additional books in this series can be found on Nova's website under the Series tab.

Additional e-books in this series can be found on Nova's website under the e-book tab.

SURGERY - PROCEDURES, COMPLICATIONS, AND RESULTS

MINIMALLY INVASIVE SURGERY FOR PITUITARY ADENOMA

METHEE WONGSIRISUWAN

NOVA BIOMEDICAL

New York

Library of Congress Cataloging-in-Publication Data

ISBN: 978-1-63482-766-9

Library of Congress Control Number: 2015945234

Published by Nova Science Publishers, Inc. † New York

Contents

Preface

When handling the pituitary adenoma, surgical avoidance is the preferable choice for the patient. However, if surgery is the only available option, a minimally invasive approach is the most preferred option for every patient. "Minimally invasive neurosurgery" has been the major development in neurosurgical specialty over the last decade. This development resulted from the innovation of many sophisticated surgical instruments combined with the usage of highly precise image guidance systems. However, neurosurgeons must understand the related anatomy and also be able to correlate important neurovascular structures with their boundaries. These are a great help to both the patient and the neurosurgeon. One of the great advantages of a minimally invasive approach is the patient's satisfaction gained from small or the altogether absent incision during the surgery. The anatomical knowledge of the gland and the relevant anatomy (i.e., major vessels, optic apparatus, nasal cavity, and paranasal sinuses) will optimize the neurosurgeon's ability to perform well. A properly planned treatment will allow surgeons perfect and comfortable results of pituitary management.

The major portion of this book will be devoted to the relevant anatomy, operative detail, approach selection, handling and how to avoid the complications including the future of minimally invasive treatment for the pituitary adenoma, especially robotic surgery. I hope that this book benefits any neurosurgeon who is involved in pituitary adenoma surgery and contributes to the evolution of minimally invasive modalities in pituitary adenoma surgery.

I would like to express my deepest gratitude to my wife *Surinya* and my only son *Siriwong*, for their tolerance and acceptance of losing our common time, spent writing for the completion of this book. Also, I would like to extend major thanks to Dr. Max Jitraphongsathorn and Dr. Suphakij Phimolthares for helping with my English-language review.

Methee Wongsirisuwan

Abstract

The pituitary gland is a very small sized gland, which plays an important role in regulating human wellbeing by controlling many activities of other hormone-secreting glands. It is embedded in a midline, bony hollow of the cranial base and is surrounded by vital structures (e.g., optic apparatus, cavernous sinuses, internal carotid arteries, and cranial nerves that control extraocular muscles). Adenoma of this gland is a challenging problem for neurosurgeons. Some are best managed with medication alone, but some are more responsive to surgery. Numerous refinements in surgical approaches to the pituitary gland have been proposed for decades. Advancements in modern surgical equipment and state-of-the-art technology of highly precise tools have given neurosurgeons a new, minimally invasive approach. Since the era of image-guided surgery, neurosurgeons were offered many chances in innovating high precision surgical techniques via a very small incision or no incision at all. Patients received many benefits from the so-called minimally invasive surgery, particularly less side effects with greater patient comfort. Better outcome, little or no scarring, and lower complication rates of pituitary adenoma surgery resulted from little tissue manipulation by cutting-edge technology. However, the revolutionized pituitary surgery is still going ahead. Starting with the microscopic era, followed by image-guidance and then by endoscopic maneuver, all of these give neurosurgeons a streamlined, multidisciplinary approach in treatment of the pituitary adenoma. Another groundbreaking development in minimally invasive treatment for pituitary adenoma is robotic surgery. Robotic surgery of pituitary adenoma offers a wide range of treatment: passive, semiactive, active robots, and remote manipulators. Some of them are non-invasive alternatives to surgery such as Gamma Knife®, LINAC, Cyberknife®; they provide pain-free, non-surgical alternative treatment for surgically complex and invasive adenomas or inoperable patients. The era of robotic surgery is going to innovate pituitary glands surgery; as a technique, it is to become the gold standard treatment. Future progress will turn minimally invasive surgery into non-invasive treatment of pituitary adenoma sooner or later.

Author Contact Information

Dr. Assist. Prof. Methee Wongsirisuwan, MD
Division of Neurosurgery
Rajavithi Hospital
2 Phayathai Rd., Rhajathevi,
Bangkok 10400, Thailand
Email: mathee@hotmail.com

Chapter I

General Background

The pituitary gland is a very small organ, found in midline at the base of the brain (Figure 1). The most common abnormality of this gland is caused by abnormal cell division resulting in pituitary adenoma. Pituitary adenomas are slow growing tumors that constitute about 15-20% of all intracranial tumors. Almost all pituitary adenomas are benign in origin. However, benign pituitary adenomas can cause many significant problems and affect many vital structures around their boundaries. The adenomas usually originate from the sella turcica, and then often grow into the walls of the sella turcica themselves. Blood vessels, cranial nerves, and meninges can be invaded by the adenomas, which are more challenging for the neurosurgeons who want to get rid of them. Pituitary adenomas can be divided in 2 subgroups based on the size:

(1) *Microadenomas*: tumors with a maximum diameter smaller than 1 centimeter (cm) are classified as microadenomas. Because of these small sizes, the tumors have less compressive symptoms but they can cause many hormonal symptoms. In the case of non-producing adenomas, they are usually not detected until they grow large enough to have compr-essive symptoms.

(2) *Macroadenomas*: tumors with a maximum diameter larger than 1 cm are classified as macroadenomas. Most of the patients with macroadenomas will come to the hospital with problems of compressive signs and symptoms created by the mass effect of the adenomas themselves. One of the most common symptoms is visual deterioration because of optic

apparatus compression by the adenoma. However, hormonal disturbances can also be detected in this subgroup.

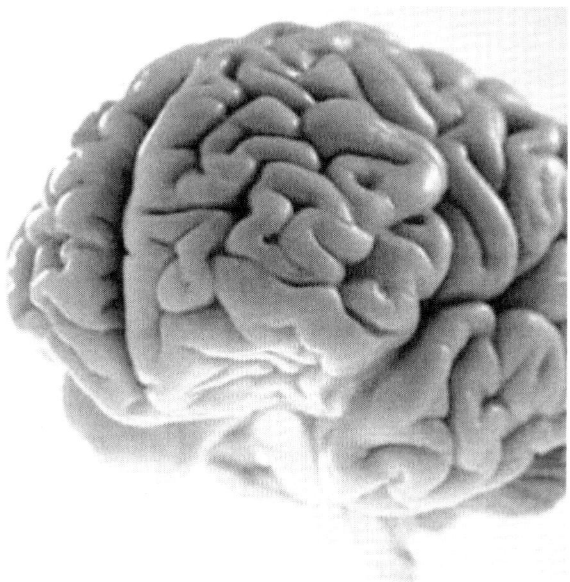

Figure 1. Pituitary gland: the master gland that controls several hormonal glands located beneath the brain.

Another pituitary adenomas' classification is based on whether the tumor makes excessive hormones or not. If they produce too much hormone, then they are called functional or producing adenomas. On the other hand, if no excessive hormone is produced they are called non-functional or non-producing adenomas. The type of hormone produced from the adenoma depends on its cell type. The most common functional adenomas are the prolactin-producing adenomas (or the so-called prolactinomas). The other functional adenomas are growth hormone-producing adenomas, thyrotropin-producing adenomas (TSH), gonadotropin-producing adenomas (LH and FSH), and corticotropin producing-adenomas (ACTH). However, some adenomas can produce more than one type of hormone. Patients with producing adenomas usually visit doctors in the early stages because of the signs and symptoms of hormonal disturbance. Non-producing adenomas are usually detected late and come with compressive signs and symptoms resulting from their large size (macroadenoma).

With the best of current medical knowledge, the etiology of pituitary adenomas are yet unknown, so the best way to handle them is to identify them as early as possible to ensure the best treatment. MRI seems to be the best modality to identify the adenomas but unfortunately, non-producing adenomas may be less sensitive to diagnosis at an early stage. However, new technology of high magnetic field MRI may alleviate this problem in the future.

Chapter II

Treatment Options

Two important factors for judgment of modalities of treatment of the adenoma are size and extension of them (micro- or macro-adenoma, structural invasion especially the optic apparatus) and hormonal production (functional or non-functional adenoma). Medical treatment, radiosurgery, and surgery are the standard available options in handling these pituitary adenomas. In some cases, combined treatments are used with excellent results. For example, for a large one, surgery is usually the first option to reduce the size of the tumor, followed by radiosurgery for tumor control. A team including internal medicine, endocrinologist, neurologist, oncologist, and a neurosurgeon should participate and discuss the best treatment options for the patient.

Chapter III

Historical Aspects for Pituitary Adenoma Surgery

Surgery seems to be the best available option for handling pituitary adenomas, especially those that invade surrounding structures, e.g., the optic apparatus and the internal carotid artery. Over the last century, the surgery has evolved from a large craniotomy toward a smaller one (called "Keyhole") or "no craniotomy" at all.

The pterional approach is commonly employed in many areas of neurosurgery especially for the anterior and the middle cranial fossa. This technique was designed and popularized by Yasargil in the early 1970s (Figure 2). Known as the father of modern neurosurgery and neurosurgery's man of the century, he summarized the brain characteristic as "The brain actually is not like a single organ. It's like the country. There are many organs. And each one a city, like St. Louis. There's a vascular organ. An endocrine organ. An immunological organ. All in the brain." He innovated approaches in neurosurgery, and also developed many neurosurgical instruments such as the Leyla self-retaining adjustable brain retractor, aneurysm clip, and the floating microscope. Briefly, this approach begins with the removal of the frontotemporal bones together with the greater wing of the sphenoid bone and followed by the transsylvian dissection to gain space deep behind the hallway (Sylvian path). When neurosurgeons come along this hallway, they can release cerebrospinal fluid (CSF) to gain more brain relaxation by opening the basal cistern [1]. With this approach, pituitary adenoma surgery can be easily performed. The subfrontal, retroorbital, prechiasmatic, chiasmatic, sellar, suprasellar, prepontine, and upper part of clival area can be seen clearly with this approach. In complex cases, such as invasive lesions around cavernous sinus, neurosurgeons can modify this approach to the extended pterional approach that more space should be gained through this procedure. Sometimes this can also be combined with an orbitozygomatic osteotomy to provide wider space for complex skull base lesions. This approach minimizes brain retraction and lessens the unnecessary iatrogenic brain damage. Multidirectional view from various extensions can allow safer manipulation during the entire operation. With the many advantages described, pterional craniotomy has been considered a standard approach for many neurosurgical procedures, including pituitary adenoma surgery, for decades. However, new operative instruments and techniques are always being developed. In the same way, neurological surgery is not the exception. Minimally invasive brain surgery is continually being developed; in the era of microscopic development followed by the endoscopic era, many neurosurgical procedures have been shifted from conventional surgery to minimally invasive surgery. Summarized by P. Grunert, evolution in minimally invasive neurosurgical techniques can be classified into four neurosurgical fields:

(1) Localization of intracerebral lesions and eloquent cortical areas,
(2) Transsphenoidal approach to the pituitary adenomas,
(3) Endoscopic treatment of hydrocephalus,
(4) Functional stereotaxic neurosurgery [2].

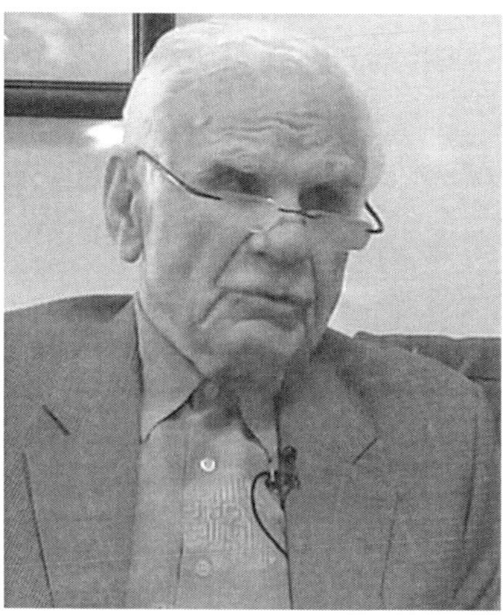

Figure 2. Gazi Yasargil: Neurosurgery's Man of the Century (1950-1999), Father of Modern Neurosurgery.

However, development of endoscopic surgery required innovative design of new endoscopic instruments and required operative techniques that are different from standard conventional surgery. Along with the development of endoscopic surgery, neuronavigation and other image guidance systems were innovated to facilitate improvement of the minimally invasive concept. These modern imaging techniques emerged with many new possibilities for neurosurgical procedures. High-precision surgical guidance minimizes high fatal-risk procedures and maximizes patient safety. The state-of-the-art of surgical navigation enables neurosurgeons to get into the deep space, which was formerly the blind spot during surgery. Axel Perneczky is the one who deserves the merits in endoscopic neurosurgery (Figure 3). He invented many specialized neurosurgical tools especially for minimally invasive techniques, and made surgery safer and more effective. His excellent skills and innovative ideas led him to become the driving force behind the modern era of minimally invasive neurosurgery. Minimally invasive techniques minimized iatrogenic trauma during surgery resulting in less postoperative morbidity. The minimally invasive neurosurgery comprised not only endoscopic surgery, but also included an image-guidance system, workstation, and 3D-microscope. His great effort created the new concept in minimally invasive neurosurgery, later named the "Keyhole concept." Through a small craniotomy, deep-seated structures can be manipulated safely.

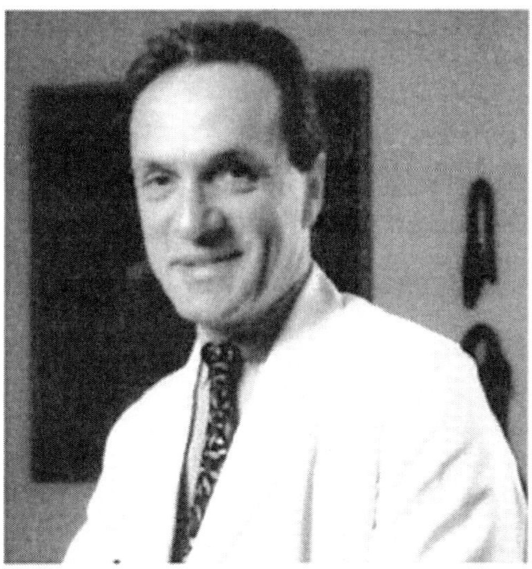

Figure 3. Axel Perneczky.

There are still certain diseases that require standard or conventional surgery, such as very large complex skull base tumors or swollen brain conditions, however, most neurosurgical procedures nowadays can be treated with some aspects of minimally invasive technique. The best options should be individualized to the patient's diagnosis and the overall condition. Pituitary adenoma surgery may be the best example in gaining the advantage of minimally invasive concept. Surgical approaches to the pituitary area have undergone numerous refinements over decades. With the introduction of the microscope followed by the image guidance system and finally the endoscopic innovation, minimally invasive pituitary surgery is claimed as the new standard procedure instead of the pterional approach. A brightness and clarity of vision from endoscope/microscope combined with the precise image guidance system increases the ability to explore this deep-seated tumor with better results. Most of pituitary adenoma patients can be discharged within a few days after the operation and can resume their normal daily life quite early.

Chapter IV

Minimally Invasive Pituitary Adenoma Surgery

Minimally invasive pituitary adenoma surgery can be classified into 2 modalities:

(1) Endoscopic endonasal transsphenoidal approach (EETA)
(2) Keyhole supraorbital approach (KSA)

Both techniques enable neurosurgeons to remove tumors through a small opening, nostrils for EETA and a keyhole craniotomy for KSA. With EETA, neurosurgeons perform the surgery by using a rigid endoscope equipped with a high-resolution camera and a very intense light (usually Xenon). With KSA, neurosurgeons perform the surgery using a sophisticated microscope through a small skull opening, usually over the supraorbital area. EETA enables neurosurgeons to access areas of the brain that cannot be reached with conventional surgery through the natural pathways (nostrils) without any visible incision. It has great benefit compared to the traditional microscopic trans-sphenoidal approach. EETA also gives neurosurgeons a superior exposure and better view, allowing a better removal under direct vision. This approach avoids unnecessary brain exposure and manipulation, which are the main cause of postoperative iatrogenic brain damage. However, KSA has more advantages over EETA especially when the tumor has spread far laterally into the cavernous sinuses. In some cases, neurosurgeons will use the endoscope as an assisted instrument in KSA. This endoscope-assisted micro neurosurgery can improve the outcome and success rate for the treatment of extensive pituitary adenoma.

Endoscopic Endonasal Transsphenoidal Approach (EETA)

Transsphenoidal surgery is one of the most common procedures used to remove pituitary adenoma for decades. Neurosurgeons have used microscopes as a tool to provide a light source for clearer vision at the base of the surgical field. However, the limitations of the microscope are a blind spot because the light cannot pass through the narrow passage. Since early in the 1960s, there was an attempt to use the endoscope as a supplement to transsphenoidal transseptal surgery. So, in the early phase of endoscopic transsphenoidal surgery, the endoscope was only used as an adjunct to microscopic transsphenoidal surgery. The endoscope reveals more details in the blind spot area such as the undersurface of the optic nerve or chiasm and the posterior surface of the internal carotid artery. This technique is called "*Endoscope-Assisted Microneurosurgery*," which means that the endoscope will be used for a short period. With this technique, both microscope and endoscope will help each other due to their different optical properties. The microscope is superior to the endoscope due to its 3-dimensional vision, but the endoscope is better than the microscope when neurosurgeons want more details in the deep and narrow space and also in the blind spot area. However, when neurosurgeons gain more experience with endoscopic handling, the advantages of the endoscope are clearly seen. Together with this, many new endoscopic instruments were innovated to support neurosurgeons during the operation. Finally, "*Pure Endoscopic Endonasal Surgery*" was proposed as a new option for pituitary adenoma surgery. Despite EETA has some limitations as compared to the traditional microscopic transsphenoidal approach such as lack of a three-dimensional view, however EETA still offers many advantages especially a very close-up view of the relevant anatomy including panoramic vision of the surgical field. Patients after EETA usually have less postoperative nasal discomfort. With a remarkable evolution of these technologies, the collaboration between neurosurgeons and ENT surgeons with many innovations in reconstruction techniques, pure endoscopic endonasal surgery is now becoming the gold standard approach for pituitary adenomas.

However, the endoscope's technique requires more skill and there is a steep learning curve. Most neurosurgeons are more familiar with microscopic skills than endoscopic skills. The first attempt seems to be the most difficult part of endoscopic pituitary adenoma removal for everyone. In order to have this special skill, neurosurgeons must know all details about anatomy and radiology related to the nasal cavity, paranasal sinus, and the skull base. The fastest way to get more endoscopic experience is team approach with the otolaryngologist (ENT). Due to the fact that ENT surgeons have better knowledge and familiarity of the anatomy of the nose and the paranasal sinuses than neurosurgeons, and vice versa for the sellar and parasellar anatomy. So, it is to the benefit of patients if both surgeons work together.

Preoperative assessment and patient preparation are also crucial steps in minimizing the unexpected events before the surgery.

Patient Preparation and Preoperative Assessment

Hypotensive technique of general anesthesia together with slightly flexion of the neck must be recommended for minimizing perioperative blood loss. Nasal preparation with high concentration adrenaline-soaked cottonoids (1:1000) for at least 5-10 minutes can significantly enlarge the nasal passage. Lidocaine plus epinephrine can decrease blood loss during the nasal phase of EETA. The patient should be placed in the supine position with the head elevated up to 20-30 degrees with slight neck flexion and the head turned towards the surgeon. In cases with a high risk of adrenal insufficiency, preoperative hormonal replacement by surgeons or endocrinologists is essential.

Anatomy of the Nasal Cavity (Figure 4)

The nostril is like the door of the nasal cavity before entering through a narrow passage that leads us to the sphenoid sinus and skull base. The nasal cavities are comprised of four walls with two openings situated in opposite directions. Anterior cranial fossa (skull base) and cribiform plates form the roof. The lateral wall is created mainly by medial wall of maxillary sinuses, lacrimal bones, ehtmoid bones, and nasal turbinates or choanae. The floor is hard palate, which divides the nasal from the oral cavity. Both nasal cavities are separated by the nasal septum, the perpendicular plate of the ehtmoid bone on the superior aspect, the vomer bone on the inferior aspect, and the quadrangular cartilage on the anterior aspect. In the deep end of this passage (posterior opening) are choanae, the sphenoid sinus, and some part of palatine bone. The middle turbinate is the largest turbinate and may be pneumatized (concha bullosa). In case of a large concha bullosa, the nasal cavity may be narrowed in the surgical corridor (nasal cavity), so partial resection may be required during the nasal phase of EETA. If we follow the superior turbinate medially, the sphenoid ostium will be seen. This ostium is the landmark for entering the sphenoid sinus, placed 1-2 cm above the choanae. Inferior to the ostium, there is an artery, which is a branch of the sphenopalatine artery. The artery sometimes causes troublesome bleeding during ostium enlarging, so it should be cauterized to avoid nasal bleeding.

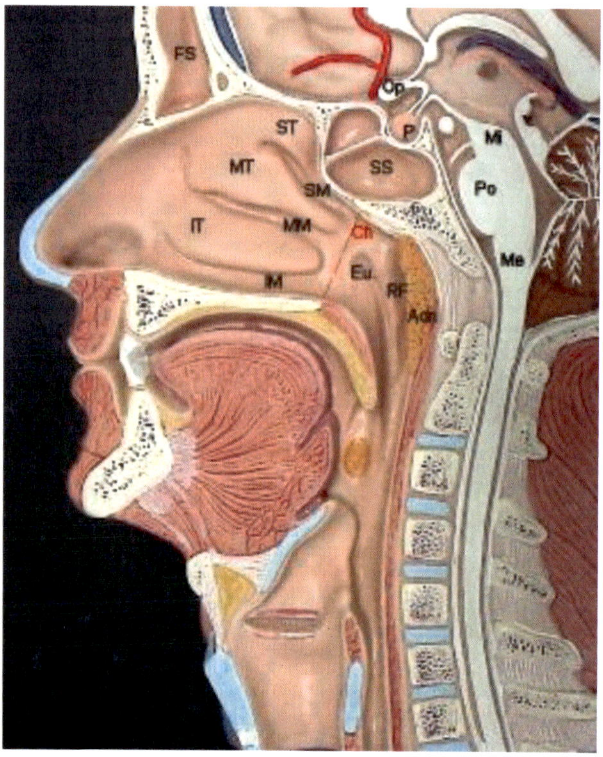

Figure 4. Lateral wall of nasal cavity (ST=Superior Turbinate, MT=Middle Turbinate, IT=Inferior Turbinate, SM=Superior Meatus, MM=Middle Meatus, IM=Inferior Meatus, SS=Sphenoid Sinus, Eu=Opening of Eustansian tube, RF=Rosenmuller fossa, Adn=Adenoid, Mi=Midbrain, Po=Pons, Me=Medulla oblongata, FS=Frontal sinus, P=Pituitary gland, Op=Optic chiasm).

The nasal septum usually divides the nasal cavities equally, but in cases with septal deviation, the larger cavity should be used first.

Anatomy of the Sphenoid Sinus

The sphenoid sinuses are highly variable. The sinuses compose two main components, sinus and bone. In most cases, there are sphenoid septums that separate the sphenoid sinus into more than one sinus. The sinus is usually composed, of two sphenoidal sinuses, the left and the right one. The sphenoid bone is not well pneumatized in every case. Actually, the degrees of this pneumatization have many variations, which should be studied with preoperative imaging. Clinically we classified it into 3 types (Figure 5).

(1) Well pneumatized (Sellar) type
(2) Partial pneumatized (Pre-sellar) type
(3) Poor pneumatized (Conchal) type

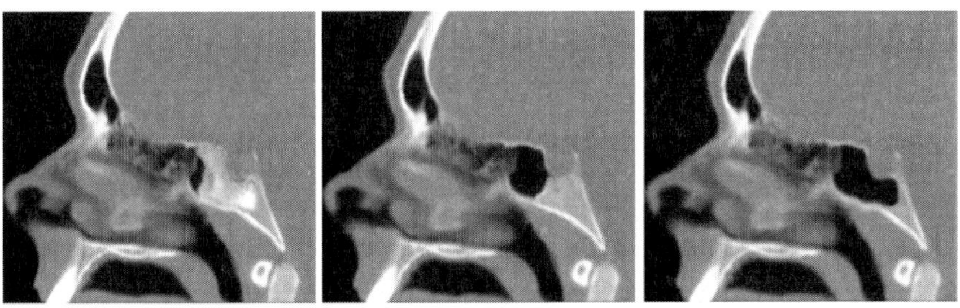

Figure 5. Sphenoid sinus (From left to right: Conchal, Pre-sellar, Sellar type).

For sellar type, the pneumatization extends from the anterior into the undersurface of the sella turcica. This type is found in most populations (70-80%). The extension of this pneumatization has great effect on the endoscopic endonasal transsphenoidal surgery. If the patient has the conchal type, then a transsphenoidal approach will be more difficult because the neurosurgeons must drill through the sphenoid sinus before entering into the sella turcica.

Another important landmark, before entering into sphenoid sinus, is the sphenoid ostium, which is usually located in the sphenoethmoidal recess. To identify this ostium (Figure 6), one must look for an area of 1.5 cm above the upper margin of the choana. The superior turbinate is also a very reliable landmark to localize the ostium, as it lies just behind the inferior aspect of the superior turbinate.

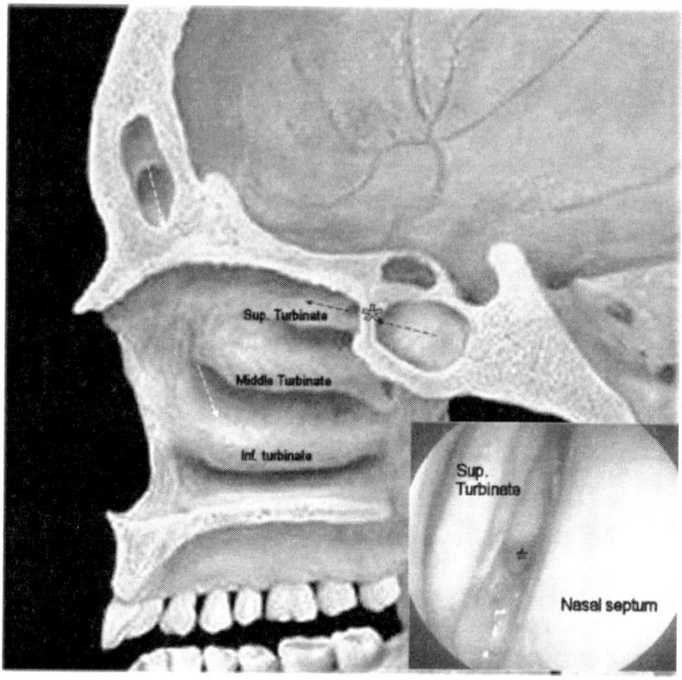

Figure 6. Sphenoid ostium (black arrow with *) and Opening of frontal sinus (white arrow).

After opening into the sphenoid sinus by enlarging the sphenoid ostium, the sphenoid septum will be shown. This is the final frontier before entering the sella turcica above. The sphenoid ostium usually represents the upper border of the anterior aspect of the sphenoid sinus, so widening the ostium is usually done by moving in a downward (inferior) direction. During this step, bleeding from the nasopalatine artery may be encountered and can be controlled easily by cauterization. When the sphenoid ostium is opened enough, the sphenoid septum will be within view. Resection of the sphenoid septum by using cutting forceps or pituitary rongeurs is mandatory before entering into the sella turcica. After complete resection of intersphenoid septum, the anterior wall of the sella turcica will present. The intersphenoid septum is rarely in the midline; it usually deviates to one side. In some cases, the septum attaches with the medial wall of the cavernous sinus where the carotid artery is embedded. Extreme caution should be used during resection of this septum to avoid injury of the internal carotid artery. If this septum deviates more laterally, it may be better to leave some part attached to the wall of the cavernous sinus. In addition to removing the septum, the sphenoid mucosa must be completely removed. Occasional bleeding from the mucosa and the sphenoid bone is usually controlled by simple monopolar cauterization. Failure to completely remove this mucosa may lead to postoperative mucocele formation. When the sphenoid sinus was completely exposed, the sella turcica floor will be seen clearly together with its bony landmark: optic protuberances and carotid protuberances.

Anatomy of Sella Turcica

Sella turcica is part of the top of the sphenoid bone. The boundary of the sella turcica comprises the lateral wall where the cavernous sinus is buried under the dura mater. The posterior wall of the sella turcica is what we called the posterior clinoid bone. The front is usually the sphenoid air cell (pneumatization of sphenoid bone). The upper part of sella turcica is its important neighbor, the pituitary stalk, and the optic apparatus.

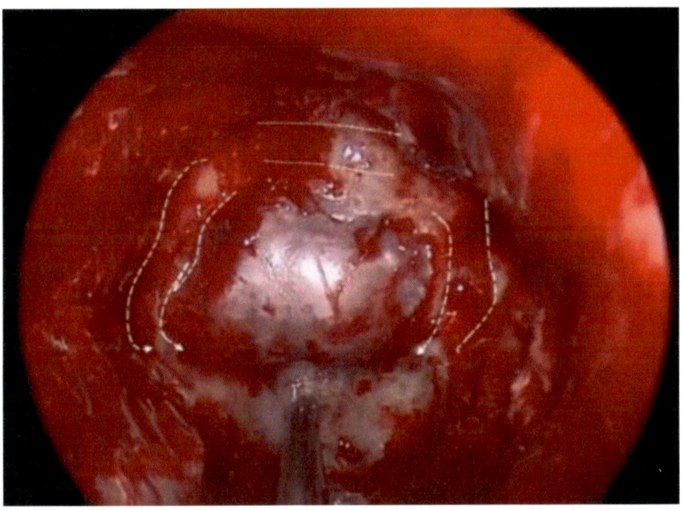

Figure 7. Carotid prominences (Double vertical arrowhead lines on left and right side) and Optic prominences (Horizontal dot lines).

The important landmark of the sella turcica lies beneath its floor or the roof of the sphenoid air cell. In this cavity, there are two downward bulges on both sides of the sella turcica called "*Carotid prominences*" (Figure 7). The prominences result from the pressure effect of the internal carotid arteries. Neurosurgeons must identify these prominences before breaking through the sella turcica floor. Failure to do this can cause disastrous and fatal events from bleeding internal carotid arteries, which are very difficult to handle. Neurosurgeons must know that in some cases, the bone that covers these prominences is dehiscent. Another way to identify this important landmark is using the small tip of a Doppler ultrasound. Medial to the carotid prominences is the "*Optic prominences*," which is the bony landmark of the optic nerve. Between the carotid and optic prominences is the area we called "*Optic-carotid recess*." This recess is also an important landmark for endoscopic approaches to the skull base. The lateral optic-carotid recess corresponds to the optic strut base and the clinoidal part of the internal carotid artery [3]. This recess is also a reliable and persistent indicator for extended transsphenoidal surgery in complex skull base cases. A careful dissection is mandatory to minimize the iatrogenic injuries to the optic apparatus and the crucial brain feeder [4].

Related Anatomy during EETA

Like microscopic transsphenoidal surgery, we can classify the approach into 3 consecutive phases.

(1) Nasal phase
(2) Sphenoid phase
(3) Sellar phase

In order to avoid fatal complications, neurosurgeons must have special skill in handling the endoscope for the entire process. This skill must be trained by the mentor and practiced. Since most neurosurgeons are not familiar with the endoscopic skill, collaboration with ENT surgeons will alleviate this problem.

Nasal Phase

The nasal phase of EETA is quite different from microscopic transseptal transsphenoidal approach. Since EETA is considered minimally invasive surgery, preservation of the normal anatomical structures is the utmost concept. For a microscopic transseptal approach, the nasal septum must be fractured by the nasal speculum in every case. Fracturing the nasal septum is the process of enlarging the opening to allow enough light to pass into the base of the surgical field. Failure to do this will hinder the light from the microscope. But for EETA, the light source is at the tip of the endoscope itself. So, it is unnecessary to break the nasal septum. The endoscope is introduced through the normal pathways (both nostrils). The choice of the nasal passage to be used is selected by the size of the nasal cavity; the larger one is better. However, in some cases, with very large adenomas or an invasive one, both nostrils can be utilized for the entire operation.

The first structure that comes into view is the nasal septum and the inferior turbinate followed by the middle turbinate. In cases with nasal septum deviation, passing the endoscope through the narrow passage will limit endoscopic visualization during the entire surgery. Other than using the larger one, surgeons can perform septoplasty in conjunction with EETA.

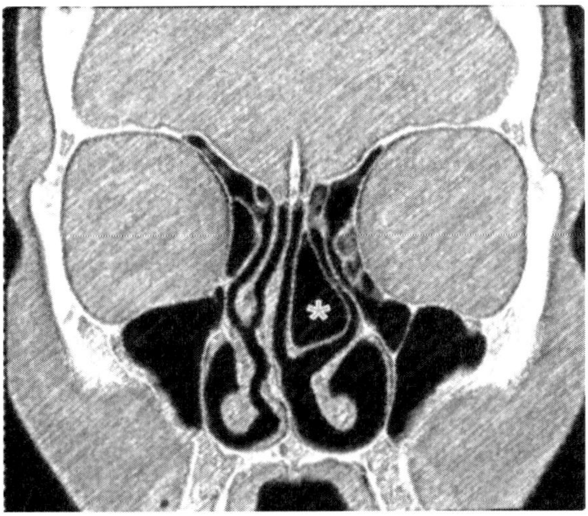

Figure 8. Concha Bullosa (*).

As the endoscope is further advanced, the next structure encountered is the middle turbinate. This turbinate is an important landmark for EETA. Superiorly, this turbinate has a close connection with the cribiform plate. Aggressive manipulation of this turbinate would damage the cribiform plate. In some cases, the middle turbinate is pneumatized (called as "Concha Bullosa") (Figure 8). If this concha bullosa obstructs the endoscope then it could be resected. However, most ENT surgeons can save this concha bullosa by using their special technique (lateralization of the middle turbinate). The middle turbinate is by far the most important landmark during this phase because it is the only pathway to the maxillary, ethmoid, and frontal sinuses. But for transsphenoidal surgery, it is unnecessary to identify all of these structures. Careful assessment of these structures from the preoperative CT scan is essential because it is a crucial factor for this nasal phase. Advancing the endoscope tip between the middle turbinate and the nasal septum, the sphenoethmoidal recess will come into view by extending between the roof of the choana and the sphenoid ostium. As mentioned above, the ostium is the entrance of the sphenoid sinus. In most cases, we can use the roof of the choana as a good reference to the ostium. Failure in identifying this natural door can cause reluctance in entering the sella turcica.

In cases of severe mucosal edema from chronic sinusitis or allergy, this ostium may not be able to be viewed. So, fluoroscopic guidance or neuronavigation can confirm the reach of the sphenoid sinus.

Sphenoid Phase

This phase begins by identifying the sphenoid ostium. As previously mentioned, the ostium is the door of the sphenoid sinus. To enter into the sinus, the ostium must be enlarged using a diamond tipped burr or the circular cutting punch (Stammberger by STORZ). The two ostiums (left and right) should be opened simultaneously to create room for the next sellar step. After enlarging the sphenoid ostium and breaking the sphenoid septum, the important landmarks such as sellar floor, clivus, planum sphenoidale, carotid prominences, and optic prominences will be exposed. Identifying the optic-carotid recess must not be forgotten, as it is a landmark for the identification of the optic nerve and the internal carotid artery. After completion of these important structures, then the sphenoid septum (Figure 9) should be resected before entering into the sella turcica. In order to avoid serious bleeding from cavernous sinuses, special care during this resection is essential because the sphenoid septum may be strongly attached with cavernous sinus walls. To gain total tumor removal, wide exposure of the sphenoid sinus is essential.

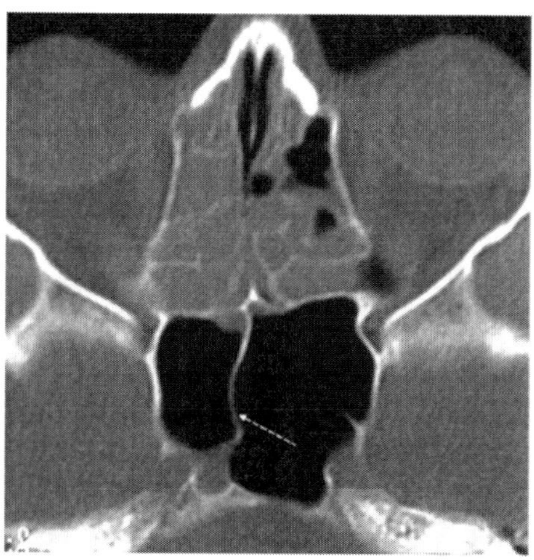

Figure 9. Sphenoid septum (arrowhead).

Sellar Phase

Before entering into the sellar, the surgeon must open the sellar floor. For less experienced neurosurgeons, confirmation of the sellar floor is mandatory. The C-arm fluoroscope or the neuronavigator is useful. In such a large macroadenoma, with high pressure to the surrounding structures, the sellar floor is usually eroded by the long-standing pressure. It can be easily broken by applying light pressure using a suction tip or a bony dissector. In case of a microadenoma or the conchal type of sphenoid sinus, a high-speed microdrill is used to open this floor. Don't use much force to break down the sellar floor because there is a possibility of carotid injury. It will be safer to start opening the sellar in the midline between the optic protuberances and the carotid bulges, which is usually a very thin bone from the pressure effect of the adenoma. Once the sellar floor is opened, then it can be enlarged using a Kerrison rongeur or Stammberger punch. The amount of the exposure depends on the size and the extension of the adenoma. Usually, the exposure will be limited laterally by the cavernous sinus, superiorly by the tuberculum sella and inferiorly by the clivus. In case of optic nerve compression, one can drill out the planum sphenoidale. Another tip to avoid the carotid artery and the cavernous sinus injury is midline drilling with neuronavigator guidance. In case of non-invasive pituitary adenoma, the extension of the sellar opening is usually limited by the important bony structures, the carotid prominences laterally, the planum sphenoidale above, and the clivus below.

After completion of all three consecutive phases, then the dura mater covering the adenomas should be presented and ready for the next intracranial step.

Intracranial Step

During this step, a team with four hands (neurosurgeon and ENT surgeon) is better than a two-hands' operation (neurosurgeon and endoscopic holder or neurosurgeon alone).

Dural incision is made better by a retractable sickle knife. There are four boundaries that limit the dural opening:

(1) Superior: superior intercavernous sinus (may be absent)
(2) Inferior: inferior intercavernous sinus (may be absent)
(3) Lateral: cavernous sinus and its contents especially internal carotid artery.

Failure to use the sharp dissection may lead to disastrous events, especially bleeding from the cavernous sinus and the carotid artery. Occasional bleeding from the cut ends of the dura can be controlled by bipolar cauterization. To enable this cauterization, it is wise to leave a thin rim of the dura away from the bony edge.

Tumor Removal

Once the dura is incised, the intrasellar lesion will be in view and be removed by curettage and suction aspiration similar to the microscopic transseptal transsphenoidal approach. In such a large macroadenoma, the tumor usually herniates through the defect immediately. After collecting this specimen for further pathologic report, the remaining intrasellar mass is removed by ring curettes and suction aspiration, using currettes, suction tubes, suction currettes, and endoscopes of varying diameters and angulation. It is possible to completely remove the microadenoma by identifying a cleavage plane of the adenoma pseudocapsule for an "en bloc" removal. A 0 degree endoscope is usually utilized as a main instrument, but if the surgeon wants to inspect the sellar cavity after tumor removal then the 30-45 degree endoscope could be helpful.

During tumor removal, all attempts should be used to preserve the normal pituitary gland and its stalk as much as possible. Failure to preserve the normal gland or the pituitary stalk will lead to permanent damage of this gland.

At the end of the tumor removal, the diaphragmatic sella and the arachnoid membrane will come into view and descend downward to the endoscope. This indicates the superior margin of the tumor and is the sign of the complete removal. Various degrees of the endoscopes should be used to completely inspect around the corners to ensure that there is no pituitary adenoma left. Gentle handling of the suction and the curettes is mandatory to avoid arachnoid tear. Suction aspiration near the diaphragmatic sella should be restricted to preserve this arachnoid and prevent postoperative CSF leakage.

It is also noted that the vision during EETA is much different from the microscopic transsphenoidal approach. For EETA, there are two main obstacles.

(1) Loss of binocular vision (loss 3D)
(2) Loss of bimanual manipulation

For binocular vision loss, this seems to be the big problem during the first few experiences of the operation. After gaining a high learning curve, binocular vision or monocular vision is not a big deal anymore. This obstacle will fade after the launching of the 3D endoscope. About bimanual manipulation, this problem is the endoscope must be held in one hand of the surgeon at all times. So, only one hand is left for the manipulation. To alleviate this problem, the endoscopic holder is the answer. But if the surgeon and an assistant with endoscopic skill do the operation, then a "three-hand" technique can be used. The assistant will hold the endoscope in order to give the surgeon the possibility of working with bimanual dissection.

Bleeding Control

The hazards and pitfalls of EETA can be anticipated with experience and knowledge of the sellar anatomy. The ability to control arterial bleeding is very important in attaining a satisfactory outcome.

Usually the pituitary adenoma itself does not cause severe bleeding. Occasional bleeding is always controlled by saline irrigation, hemostasis material, or bipolar cauterization. Most severe bleeding complications occur from iatrogenic injury to neighbor structures. The intercavernous sinuses (Figure 10) may be traumatized during the operation, however it can be controlled by light pressure and packing during the operation.

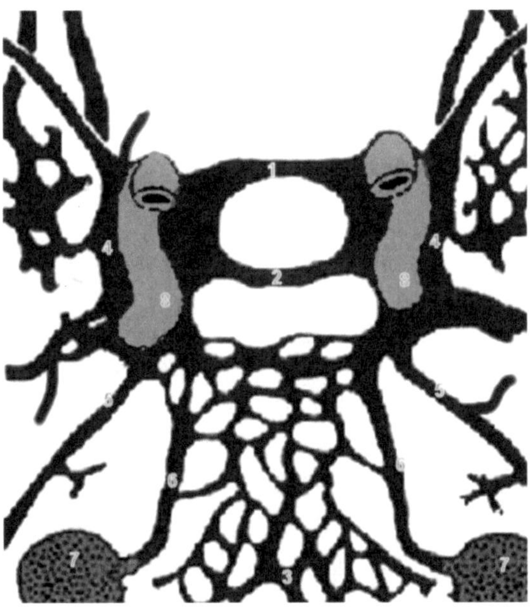

Figure 10. Cavernous sinus and its tributaries: 1. Anterior intercavernous sinus 2. Posterior intercavernous sinus 3. Basilar venous plexus 4. Cavernous sinus 5. Superior petrosal sinus 6. Inferior petrosal sinus 7. Transverse sinus 8. Carotid artery.

The most fatal hemorrhagic complications during transsphenoidal surgery usually result from injury to the internal carotid artery. Although it is rare, when it occurs it may lead to permanent disability or death. Many surgical techniques are proposed to control this fatal event. The cervical carotid artery may be compressed by the assistant to give the surgeon enough time to handle bleeding. Hemostasis material to control bleeding such as Surgicel® (Johnson & Johnson), Gelfoam® (Codman), hemostasis matrix like Floseal® or Fibrin glue may be helpful. With hybrid operating theatre, an endovascular occlusion can be used. However, the best way to handle this fatal problem is extreme precaution.

Sellar Repair

During tumor removal, it is mandatory to preserve the arachnoid membrane superior to the tumor, otherwise CSC leakage is unavoidable. Jugular compression applied by the anesthesiologist is usually helpful in detecting the CSF leakage. In case of significant leakage during the operation, there are many options to handle this problem. A multilayer sellar reconstruction using the abdominal fat graft (Figure 11), Gelfoam, and fibrin glue must be utilized to achieve a safe and effective sellar reconstruction. The goal of this repair is to guarantee the watertight closure (CSF leakage prevention), collapsing the dead space after tumor removal, and preventing postoperative descending of the optic apparatus into the sellar cavity. Different techniques are used to ensure the postoperative CSF leakage but one of the most well-known techniques in preventing postoperative CSF leakage is the pedicle nasoseptal flap.

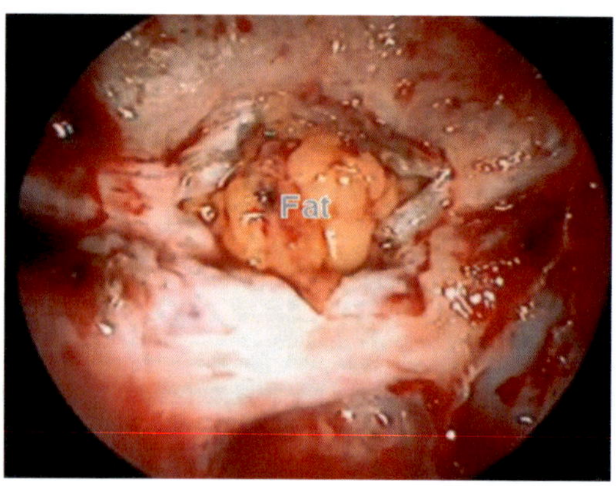

Figure 11. Abdominal fat graft was packed after complete tumor removal.

The pedicle nasoseptal flap (the Hadad-Bassegasteguy flap) is the vascular pedicle mucosal flap that is prepared during the nasal phase (Figure 12). It is made from the nasal septum mucoperichondrium and mucoperiosteum based on the nasoseptal artery (a branch of the posterior septal artery, which is a branch of the sphenopalatine artery). This flap is created in the beginning of EETA, and it is very useful in case of general skull base reconstruction after endonasal surgery. In a well-prepared case, it can cover the large anterior skull base defect. Due to its vascularized property, it is a reliable option for covering the defect. Wound healing is promoted and the incidence of CSF leakage is decreased.

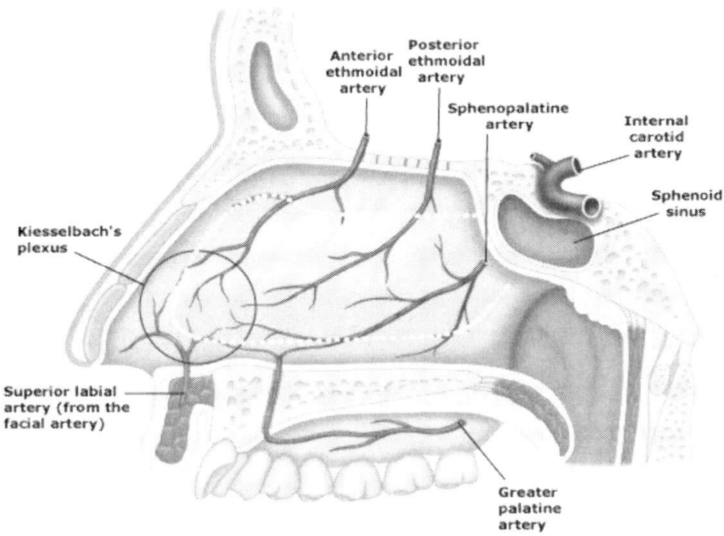

Figure 12. Nasoseptal flap (white dot line).

Reconstruction of the sellar floor with watertight dura repair is mandatory, suboptimal reconstruction with inadequate repair may potentially lead to CSF leakage, meningitis, and pneumocephalus. Therefore, reconstruction of the sellar should be carried out carefully to avoid postoperative CSF leakage.

There is a proposed grading about intraoperative CSF leakage by Esposito F. et al. [5]. The leakage can be categorized into 4 grades:

(1) Grade 0: no leakage to be observed
(2) Grade 1: small leakage without obvious diaphragmatic defect
(3) Grade 2: moderate leakage
(4) Grade 3: large diaphragmatic/dural defect

Cranial base repair is tailored to the mentioned leakage as follows:

(1) Grade 0: collagen sponge
(2) Grade 1: two-layered collagen sponge repair with intrasellar titanium mesh buttress or intrasellar fat graft (in case of large intrasellar dead space) ± Bioglue® (Cryolife, Inc., Atlanta, GA)
(3) Grade 2: intrasellar and sphenoid sinus fat grafts with collagen sponge overlay and titanium buttress ± Bioglue® (Cryolife, Inc., Atlanta, GA)
(4) Grade 3: same as grade 2 with CSF diversion

In cases of large macroadenoma or with large suprasellar extension, fat grafts should be packed in the sella to prevent postoperative empty sella syndrome. Remember that the key success in prevention of CSF leakage is the arachnoid membrane. If the arachnoid membrane is intact and is reinforced by a multilayer flap then CSF leakage will no longer be encountered. In case of arachnoid tear over the sellar area, repair or reinforcement with biomaterial substance such as fibrin glue, graft, or fat is essential. If possible, in every case, reconstruction of the sellar floor by autologous bone graft/synthetic material (titanium mesh graft) is strongly suggested. In cases with the extended approach, a balloon to reinforce the skull base is useful to prevent the postoperative migration of the graft or the material. However, the position of the balloon must be in the proper place to ensure that there is no compression over the critical organs, especially the optic apparatus or the internal carotid artery.

Nasal Passage Repair

Before leaving from the tunnel, if the middle turbinate is displaced laterally then it must be replaced in its original position. Failure to reposition this turbinate may cause postoperative maxillary sinusitis. All nasal bleeding should be easily stopped by light pressure without nasal packing. However, some ENT surgeons prefer to pack the nasal cavity with Merocel® nasal packing.

Extended Approach for Invasive Pituitary Adenoma

Some pituitary adenomas extend beyond the sella turcica into the cavernous sinus and optic canal. In order to achieve total removal, more of the skull base must be resected by extended endoscopic transsphenoidal approach. Cappabianca and his team summarized the transplanum approach very well. In this approach, the posterior part of the planum sphenoidale must be removed using a slim type of high-speed drill (diamond-tipped microdrill). The important anatomical landmark of the planum sphenoidale sits on both sides (far lateral) called "the protuberances of the optic nerves." Care should be taken to avoid heat injury from the high-speed drill. It is highly recommended to leave a thin leaf of bone attached with the optic nerve. This bone should be removed later by a small Kerrison bone punch or other specially designed instruments.

For pituitary adenoma with a cavernous sinus extension, the surgery will be more complicated because the cavernous sinus contains important neurovascular structures: internal carotid artery, oculomotor nerve, trochea nerve, ophthalmic and maxillary division of trigeminal nerve, and abducen nerve. During the sphenoid phase, the bone that covers the cavernous sinus (lateral sphenoid wall) must be drilled off with special care. Once the carotid protuberance comes into view then it reaches the intracavernous portion of the internal carotid artery. Medialization of the internal carotid artery will expose the important neurovascular structures. If surgeons are not familiar with this approach, an ultrasound Doppler probe can be helpful for identifying the intracavernous sinus portion of the internal carotid artery, thus allowing a safer opening of the dura.

If pituitary adenoma extends beyond the sellar down to the clivus (called "invasive pituitary adenoma), then the posterior skull base approach (transclival approach) must be utilized. First done by drilling out the inferior part of the sellar floor to reach the superior part of the clivus. The opening of the clivus should be done in a cranio-caudal direction using a diamond burr plus a Kerrison punch. The vomer and the floor of the sphenoid sinus must be removed completely to achieve full exposure of the entire clivus. The landmark for lateral limit of the drilling is the vidian nerve. If we follow this nerve, it will guide us to the anterior genu of the horizontal segment of the internal carotid artery. Careful inspection of this nerve can reduce the risk of the injury of the internal carotid artery during drilling. It should also be kept in mind that particular attention must be paid to drilling out the clivus; a thin leaf of bone must be preserved and removed later by Kerrison rongeurs. Normally, the dura attached with the clivus is usually covered by the venous plexus, so special care must be taken during dural opening. Once the dura is completely opened, the brainstem together with the basilar artery and the oculomotor nerves will be completely exposed and ready for further dissection.

The important issue to be kept in mind is that the wider the opening is, the higher the risk of postoperative CSF leak. If the case needs extensive approach by drilling out more bone and more dural opening, then it is important to reconstruct the dura in a watertight fashion, as much as possible. A multilayer technique by restoring all the anatomic planes together with the use of fat, artificial dura, bone fragment, mucosal flap, and fibrin glue to seal the arachnoid is very important.

Usually in these extended approaches with multilayer reconstruction, it is necessary to use postoperative nasal packing for a few days. Any activities that may raise the intracranial pressure, such as nose blowing or strain related activity, are prohibited for a few weeks. If all of those recommended instructions fail to prevent or stop postoperative CSF leakage, then reoperation or the use of continuous lumbar drainage may be needed.

General Postoperative Care and Postoperative Complications

Usually, postoperative care after EETA is much as same as conventional microscopic transsphenoidal approach. The complications found in postoperative course usually results from the perioperative phase, such as CSF leakage, postoperative bleeding, nasal discomfort, etc. Better results can be achieved from skillful endoscopic usage and careful planning by the surgeons and his team.

In general, the complications can be divided into two groups: anatomical (oronasofacial, sphenoid sinus, intrasellar, suprasellar and parasellar) and endocrinological complications (anterior and/or posterior pituitary dysfunctions). The study from Gondim et al. showed that endocrinological complications occurred more frequent than anatomical complications. The most common anatomical complication is CSF leakage, whereas anterior lobe insufficiency occurred more commonly than diabetes insipidus [6].

Anatomical Complications

Nasal passage complication: Blocked nose feeling is the common sequelae after EETA resulting from the manipulation of the nasal apparatus, especially the turbinates. This symptom may last for a week but can easily be handled by medications. In an extensive approach, this symptom may last longer than simple EETA and usually resulted from extensive turbinectomies and sinus exploration. Another common nasal complication is nasal crusting which is usually associated with anosmia or loss of smell. Fortunately, these symptoms are spontaneously resolved within a few weeks. Sinusitis may occur in some cases but can easily be handled by simple medications.

Another complication related to the nasal airway is nose bleeding. Usually, this complication is related to the mucosal capillaries/arteries and can be handled using tamponade. In a very rare case, the bleeding may result from a large artery such as the sphenopalatine artery or the internal carotid artery. Epistaxis from the sphenopalatine artery may require reoperation to stop the bleeding by electrical cauterization. Massive bleeding from the internal carotid artery is the most fatal complication and demands immediate response with either reoperation or endovascular maneuver.

CSF leakage complication: One of the most common complications and maybe the most serious one is CSF leakage. The more extensive approach, the more the likelihood of this complication occurs. However, with the use of nasoseptal flap and multilayer closure technique, the incidence of this complication is now lowered. The best way to prevent this complication is in the perioperative stage by meticulous reconstruction of the sellar floor. For the postoperative period, useful instructions should be given, especially how to avoid straining, nose blowing, coughing, sneezing, and intense physical activities during the first week after the operation. After one week, the incidence of CSF leakage is very low so the patients can resume normal activity.

Endocrinological Complications

Diabetes insipidus (DI) seemed to be one of the most-encountered problems in the postoperative phase. Most of the post-pituitary surgery DI is only transient DI resulting from the manipulation, traction, or iatrogenic injury to the pituitary stalk or post-hypophyseal trauma. Fortunately, DI can be controlled by medication and is not a life threatening condition when under close supervision by endocrinologists.

The preoperative risk factors for postoperative DI as reported by Blake Charles Walker BS. et al. include histology, tumor size, post-op sodium, change in sodium, and urine output. Immediate post-operative sodium is a predictive factor for developing permanent DI [7]. As reported by Shah S and Har-EI G, the incidence of immediate DI after EETA is lower than the microscopic trans-sphenoidal approach (15% vs. 36%, respectively). They classified the incidence into short- and long-term DI. Short-term DI is defined as less than 2 weeks incidence while long-term DI is more than 6 months. The incidence of the short-term group is still lower in EETA group while the incidence of long-term DI is not significantly different [8].

The most severe endocrinological complication is pituitary apoplexy. In such a case, it can occur when there is a remaining part of the adenoma left in the sellar or suprasellar area. This situation requires immediate reoperation to save the patient from acute blindness as a result of severe optic apparatus compression.

Comparative Approach Between EETA and Traditional Microscopic Transsphenoidal Approach

The microscopic conventional transsphenoidal approach has been widely accepted for pituitary adenoma surgery for a long period. At the beginning, it was considered a minimally invasive surgery when compared with the transcranial (pterional) approach. But since the era of the endoscopic surgery, it is now considered more invasive than EETA.

For EETA, pituitary adenoma is removed through the natural pathway (nostrils), which requires no visible incision. The endoscope is passed through the nasal passageway instead of the created one via the upper gum of the mouth. As described by Cappabianca et al., EETA can be classified into three consecutive phases, the nasal, sphenoid, and sellar phases [9]. Unlike the traditional transseptal transsphenoidal approach, there is no use for a transsphenoidal retractor. Therefore, there is no destruction of the nasal septum, which is the main cause of postoperative nasal deformity and discomfort. The most critical stages are the sphenoid and sellar phases in which neurosurgeons have to identify many important landmarks, especially the carotid prominence. Failure to identify this prominence may cause internal carotid injury, which is potentially fatal. In the large series study by Arbolay et al., 278 pituitary adenomas surgeries were performed using EETA, and total removal was achieved in 92.4%. The most common complication was CSF leakage, which was encountered more frequently in cases of macroadenomas with extensive suprasellar extension requiring opening of the subarachnoid space during the dissection [10]. They stressed that watertight repair by different techniques, especially the nasoseptal flap, is mandatory. Permanent diabetes insipidus occurred in 11 patients, while four patients developed panhypopituitarism postoperatively.

A study from Joseph B., et al. reported that EETA provides more complete tumor resection and reduces complications. From their study, 75 fully endoscopic transsphenoidal operations were included in this series. Excluding hormonal symptoms, the most common presenting complaints were headache (35%) and visual symptoms (32%). Complications related to glandular injury were markedly reduced by EETA; this is reflected by the low incidence of anterior pituitary insufficiency and diabetes insipidus [11].

After study by Yang Gao et al., the rate of gross total removal (GTR) by EETA is higher than by traditional microscopic transsphenoidal approach. The rates of GTR in the endoscopic and microscopic group are 71.8% and 58.0% respectively. About CSF leakage, endoscopy appears to have a huge advantage in reconstruction because it improves visualization. However, in their study, the rate of post-operative leaks was similar (12.8% versus 12.2% for the endoscopic and microscopic groups, respectively). The main reason for this similarity may be that the improved exposure during endoscopic surgery would encourage the surgeons to extend the limits of their operation more aggressively, which may offset the minimally invasive nature of endoscopic resections and increase the rate of post-operative CSF leakage. However, EETA still decreased hospital stay and reduced observed post-operative complications (septal perforation) [12].

At present, EETA should be the first-line option for pituitary adenoma surgery. The surgical corridor using after EETA is the natural one as compared with the corridor created by breaking the normal structure after microscopic transsphenoidal approach. This is the important reason why EETA is the most minimally invasive method for pituitary adenoma surgery.

One of the reasons is that excellent visualization results from the high quality endoscope and illumination. The improved outcomes of EETA should be credited to the development of light source and endoscopes, superior illumination and visualization, and micro instruments designed especially for endoscopic surgery.

In summary, pure EETA has several advantages over microscopic transsphenoidal surgery:

- nasal septum preservation
- alleviate the blind spot
- improved visualization of important structures (close-up view) esp. carotid prominences, optic bulbs, and brain stem
- improve the ability to differentiate normal pituitary gland from the adenoma
- avoid the lip paresthesia (numbness)
- less postoperative pain and more comfortable
- less nasal airway comfortable
- more rapid recovery period

However, in order to achieve those mentioned advantages from EETA, it is important that neurosurgeons should have endoscopic skills, either by laboratory training or by collaboration with ENT surgeons.

Keyhole Supraorbital Approach (KSA)

Since 1975, the pterional approach described by Yasargil is a very remarkable approach for pituitary surgery. This approach enables total exposure of the whole frontoparietotemporal area. The opening of the entire Sylvian fissure (trans-sylvian) makes this approach quite popular in pituitary adenoma surgery. Over the past decades, since the era of "minimal invasive concept," the pterional craniotomy has undergone many developments and has been modified by several neurosurgeons, which gave rise to smaller and smaller craniotomies. Among them, the supraorbital keyhole approach (KSA) stands out.

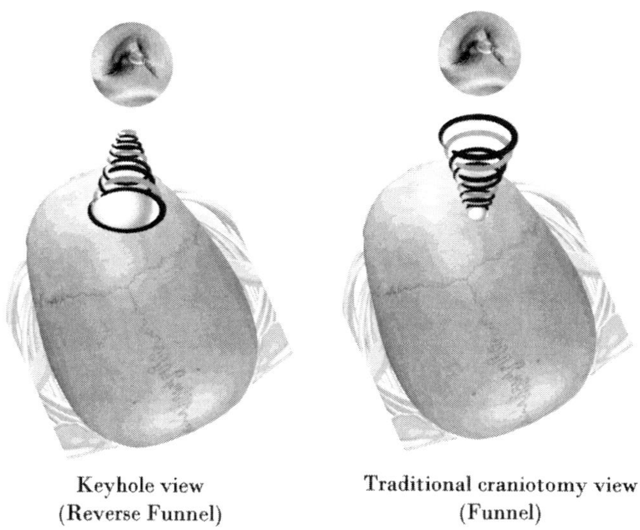

Figure 13. View after Keyhole surgery as compared with Traditional one.

Keyhole or minimally invasive surgery is a procedure of performing an operation without having to make a large incision. The named "keyhole" refers to the ability to see the entire room through the keyhole of a door. The view after the keyhole is like a reverse funnel shape whereas the view of the traditional craniotomy is a funnel shape (Figure 13). Keyhole surgery does not differ much from the traditional craniotomy except that it aims to open the incision as little as necessary – no more and no less – to achieve the surgical goals. It has to be stressed that the goal of this approach is not only to perform the smallest incision and craniotomy, but for access to adequately attack the lesions while minimizing trauma to the surrounding structures. In short, the advantage of KSA is that it required a smaller incision as compared with the traditional pterional approach. Only one small bur hole via a smaller incision carries a lower risk of iatrogenic trauma to neurovascular structures that supply the temporalis muscle. With meticulous suturing of the skin incision, KSA results in excellent cosmetic outcomes. There were many neurosurgeons who participated in the development of this approach but the one who deserves the credit that makes this approach more popular should be Axel Perneczky. He described the keyhole supraorbital craniotomy via an eyebrow skin incision very well. Not only for pituitary adenoma surgery, he also applied keyhole surgery through an eyebrow for numerous lesions such as intracranial aneurysmal surgery, craniopharyngioma, tuberculum meningioma and so on. Many textbooks about keyhole and minimally invasive neurosurgery were published worldwide. They gave us new knowledge and allowed us to upgrade the keyhole principle.

Timeline of KSA Approach

As already mentioned that the transsylvian pterional approach was accepted as the standard approach not only for pituitary adenoma surgery, but for all anterior and some middle cranial fossa lesions. However, since the concept of "less pain, less scar" surgery was introduced, all surgical procedures were shifted to "minimal invasive concept." The great leap in neurosurgical operation started with the introduction of the modern microscope. The operative techniques, modern microinstruments, and neuronavigators also supported this great leap. The great advantage of KSA is to eliminate the excessive surgical manipulation without sacrificing the surgical outcome.

Step-by-Step Surgery

After general anesthesia, the patient's head is fixed by a Mayfield three-point head holder. The positioning of the head is a very important factor. For pituitary adenoma, the tumor is usually seated in the midline with some degree of lateral extension. To allow brain relaxation with slight brain retraction, it is necessary to position the head in a slightly extended (15-20 degrees) position (Figure 14). In this position, the gravity will be the natural retractor i.e., the frontal lobe will fall away from the anterior skull base (orbital roof) by the gravity. In cases with more lateral extension, the head should be turned contralaterally to the side of the extension. With this position, the lesion will be in the same direction of the surgeon's visualization. It is recommended that the head should not be turned more than 30 degrees because most pituitary adenomas extend to both sides (Figure 13). To achieve more visualization during the surgery, the operative table can be rotated instead. Decision making about the side of the approach depends on careful preoperative planning by neurosurgeons, so it should be individually selected. Usually the key factors in choosing the side of the approach are

(1) lateral extension
(2) involvement of surrounding structures
(3) extension of frontal sinus

If both sides can be used, it is the author's opinion to operate via the right side (nondominant brain).

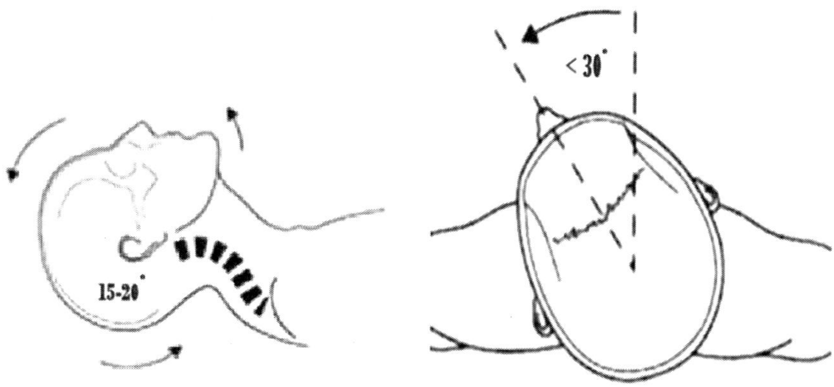

Figure 14. Optimum position for KSA in pituitary surgery.

Skin Incision

The other name of KSA is "*Eyebrow approach*" since the incision is made along the (superciliary) or within (transciliary) the eyebrow (Figure 15). There are many proposed incisions for better cosmetic results such as the incision above the eyebrow, inside or outside the eyebrow, but special care must be used to preserve the hair of the eyebrow for excellent cosmetic appearance [13]. The lateral extension of the incision depends on how much the lesion extends laterally. For medial extension of the incision, it is better to preserve the supraorbital vessels and nerves by limiting the incision medial to the supraorbital notch/foramen (Figure 16). However, in some cases, the incision may extend beyond the supraorbital notch/foramen and nerve sacrificing is unavoidable. So, the patient should be advised preoperatively that forehead numbness and asymmetry of the forehead muscle might be happened postoperatively. The skin dissection should be done in 2 consecutive steps. First, the incision is made from skin through the dermis, leaving the orbicularis oculi muscle intact. This is the first layer of the dissection. Then the dissection continues upward (superior to the eyebrow) for a few centimeters. The second layer of the dissection is begun by cutting the pericranium and the orbicularis oculi in one piece. Then the pericranium and the muscle are reflected downward (inferior). With this step, the orbicularis oculi muscle can be preserved in one piece for an excellent cosmetic result. For the lateral course, the incisions should follow the temporal line then the temporal muscle is stripped from the bony insertion and allows mobilization. After completion of the incision, the skull will be exposed and well prepared for the next important step.

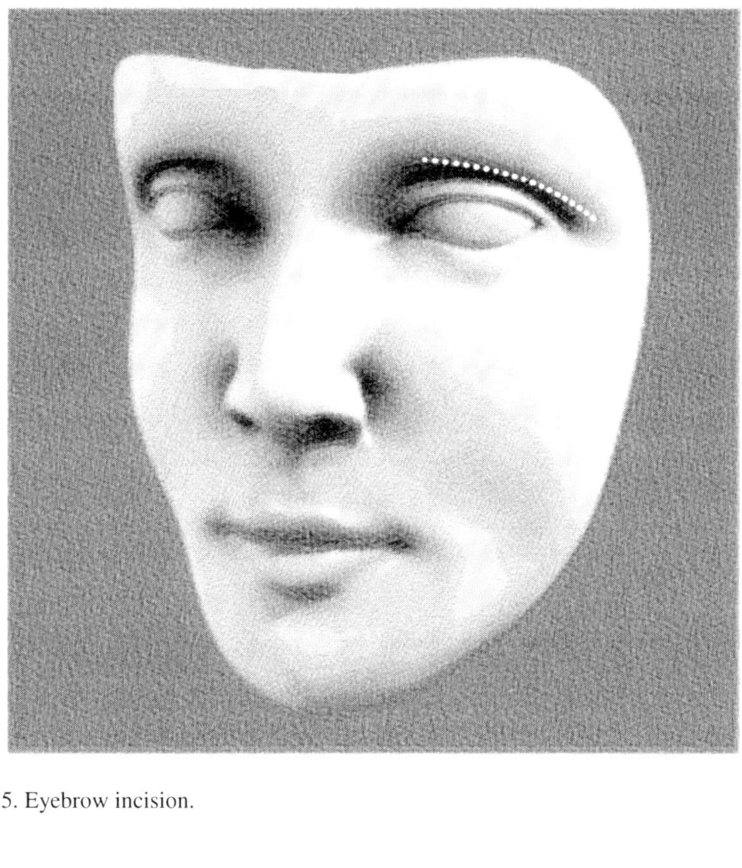

Figure 15. Eyebrow incision.

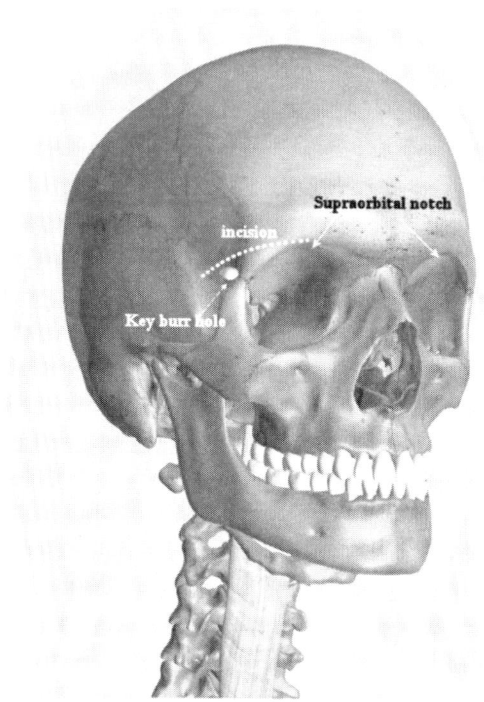

Figure 16. Relationship of Incision vs. Supraorbital notch vs. Key burr hole.

Keyhole Craniotomy

"Keyhole craniotomy" was named in this step. The skull will be opened in limited diameter (usually 3-4 cm in diameter). A single burr hole is created at the far lateral aspect of the incision close to the frontal root of the zygomatic arch (frontolateral aspect) (Figure 16). This hole is usually made by a 5 mm burr hole or by a small craniotome perforator (pediatric perforator). Special care must be utilized to preserve the dura intact during the burr. It is the standard of the author to use a pediatric perforator instead of the 5 mm burr because the standard perforator has an automatic stop mechanism, which can prevent an accidental tear of the dura and underneath the brain injury. When the key burr hole is made then the skull is ready to be opened by the high-speed craniotome. The base of the craniotomy should be made along and close to the supraorbital rim as much as possible. It is crucial to have the cutline of the bone that's close to the orbital roof to minimize frontal lobe retraction. Failure to do this will make the surgeon forcefully retract the frontal lobe during subfrontal approach, and may lead to unfavorable postoperative overretraction of the frontal lobe. Craniotomy may be made laterally from the key burr hole in more extensive cases.

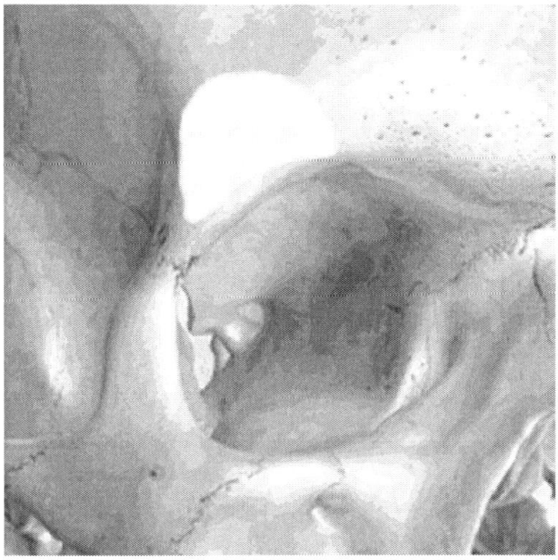

Figure 17. Keyhole craniotomy.

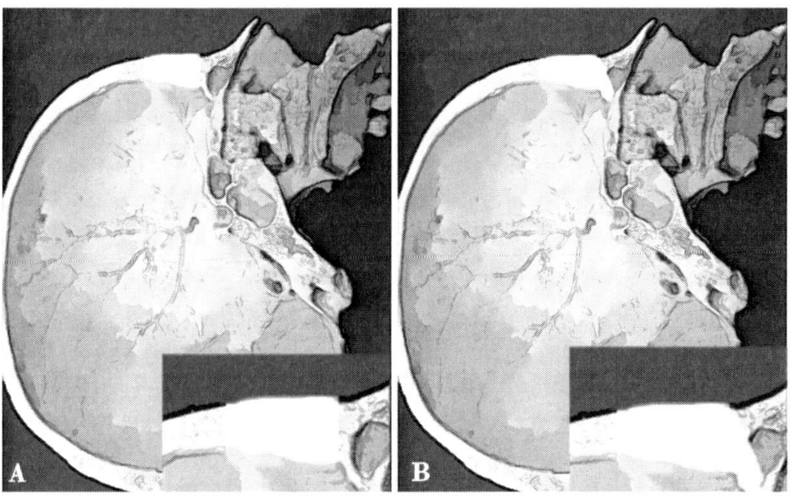

Figure 18. Before (A) and After (B) drill inner edge of orbital ridge.

Superiorly, the craniotome can be moved upward and curved over the skull to complete the opening (Figure 17). The size of the craniotomy is usually about 2-3 cm in a standard keyhole approach and 3-5 cm for more lateral extensive lesions. The smaller the craniotomy size, the harder the manipulation through the surgical procedure. In cases where the frontal sinus is broken during the craniotomy, all attempts should be made to prevent postoperative CSF leakage by watertight dural repair. Before proceeding to the next step, special care must be used to observe the orbital ridge after craniotomy. In some cases, the inner edge of the orbital ridge must be drilled off using a high-speed drill to ensure maximal visualization during the surgical procedures (Figure 18). Remember to protect the dura during drilling.

Dural Opening

Before the dural opening, the dura should be suspended to the bone edge in every case to prevent postoperative epidural hematoma. By extradural maneuver, the dura is dissected out of the orbital roof and all orbital ridges over the orbital roof (anterior cranial fossa) must be drilled off. This will also maximize the exposure and ensure clear visualization under the microscopic dissection. In elderly patients, it is more difficult to perform this step by extradural maneuver so the intradural maneuver could be performed instead, but the watertight dural repair must be ensured at the end of the operation. The dura is opened in C or D-shapes and based along the orbital rim (Figure 19). To access the lesion, the frontal lobe must be moved away from the orbital roof, but great care must be utilized by slight brain retraction after CSF drainage. In the old one, it is easier to gain access by slight retraction of the frontal lobe by brain retractors. But in the younger one, the less experienced surgeons will find that it is not easy to expose the space without frontal lobe damage. The key to this success is to release the CSF by opening the arachnoid over the frontal lobe and in some cases, mannitol usage will be helpful. After the brain is pulsated then it is time to apply the brain retractor over the frontal base. The cottonoids should be placed over the frontal lobe before applying the retractor. The operating microscope is now brought into place for a further step.

After the gentle brain retraction, the CSF comes out continuously and then the brain will be relaxed enough for further approach. More force can be applied to expose the space and the Sylvian's fissure. Conventional transsylvian dissection is done by cutting the arachnoid over the Sylvian's fissure. After enough CSF was drained out, then the routine subfrontal approach can be done easily. If the surgeons follow the Sylvian's fissure downward, the internal carotid artery (ICA) and the CSF cisterns will come into view. More CSF can be released by opening these cisterns. Now, all vital structures such as ICA, optic nerves, optic chiasm, oculomotor nerve, olfactory nerves, and pituitary adenomas can be seen clearly and ready for further lesion removal (Figure 20).

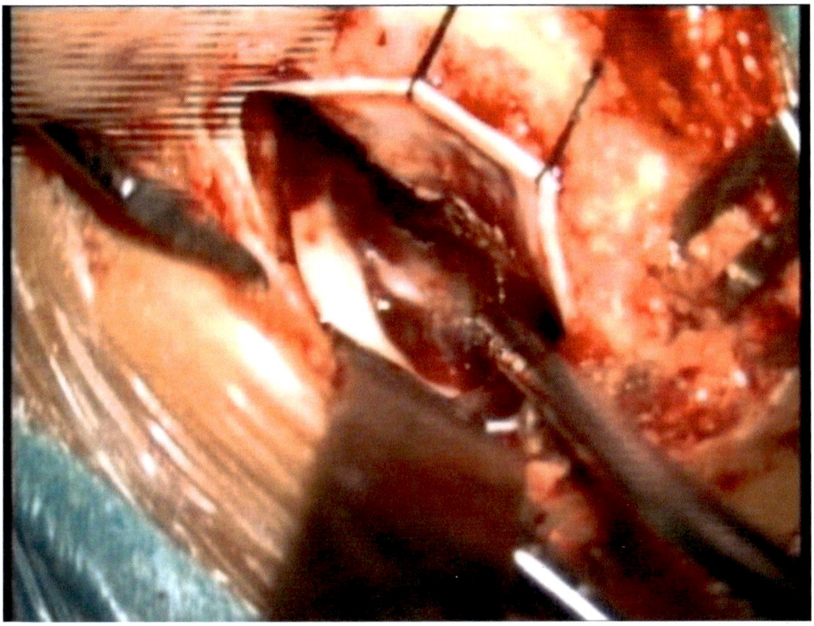

Figure 19. Dura was open in C- or D-shaped (base along with supraorbital ridge).

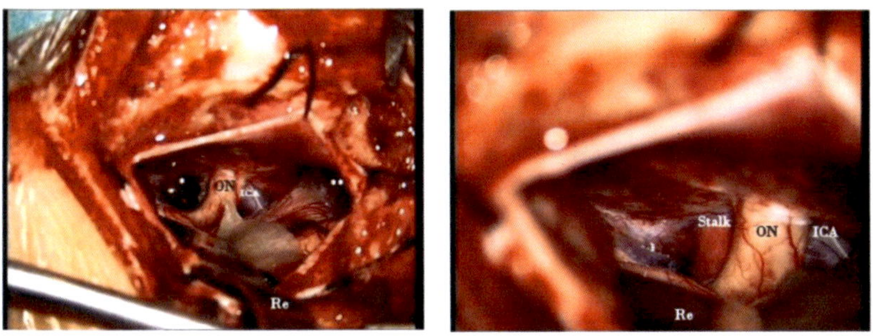

Figure 20. Direct after completion of KSA (ON=right optic nerve, ICA=right internal carotid artery, Stalk=pituitary stalk, Re=brain retractor under the frontal base, *=prechiasmatic cistern, **=Sylvian vein).

Dissection and Tumor Removal

Once all the important landmarks are identified via the subfrontal approach, the dissection can begin. Usually pituitary adenoma is a well-defined lesion; the tumor is usually contained in the thick vascularized capsule. With a combination of sharp dissection, bipolar cauterization, and microdissection techniques, the tumor can be gradually internally decompressed. After the tumor is decompressed, the surrounding structures can be identified easily, especially the internal carotid artery. In case of large pituitary adenomas, it is better to begin the incision in the capsule between both optic nerves. Bleeding from the capsule is usually controlled by simple cauterization but great care must be used to prevent the optic nerve from thermal injury during cauterization. Due to the small craniotomy and the limitation of vicinal neurovascular structures, the tumor should be removed in piecemeal fashion. In most cases, pituitary adenomas are easily suckable with less bleeding. After complete tumor removal, the tumor bed area is copiously irrigated with normal saline solution. Hemostasis is secured by simple bipolar cauterization and light pressure with the aid of Surgicele®. Special attention shall be paid to preserve the pituitary stalk from iatrogenic injury. In pituitary adenoma surgery, it is easier to preserve the stalk than in craniopharyngioma surgery. The stalk can be noticed by its remarkable appearance i.e., bright redness in color. Accurate isolation of the stalk together with gland preservation technique plays an important role in promoting postoperative recovery and avoiding postoperative endocrinological complications.

Dural Closure

The dura is closed in standard fashion. Watertight closure is imperative to prevent postoperative CSF leakage. Dural closure is facilitated by dissecting the dura free from the attached skull base. If necessary, a dural substitute or a small piece of temporalis fascia can be used to approximate the dura. Bioglue®, Fibrin glue, or another dural sealant can be used to ensure the watertight closure. Positive pressure by anesthesiologists should be done before proceeding to bone closure. If CSF still comes out, then all attempts must be made to stop CSF leakage.

Skull Fixation

Before placing the keyhole bone flap back in place, the frontal sinus must be prepared in standard fashion to prevent postoperative mucocele. To avoid the unstable fixation of bone flap and sinking skin from the wide bone seam, the skull should not be fixed by wiring method. Fixation by a circular titanium plate over the burr hole is crucial for better cosmetic appearance (Figure 21). The bone seam resulted from the bone lost during craniotomy can be filled by any injectable hydroxyapatite bone substitute or covered by titanium plates.

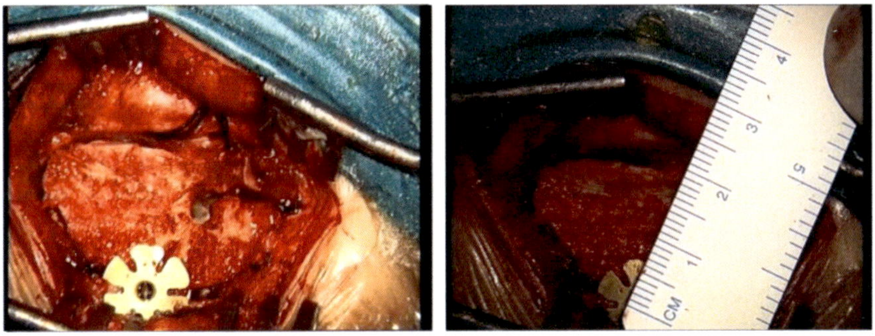

Figure 21. Skull fixation (noted the golden circular plate).

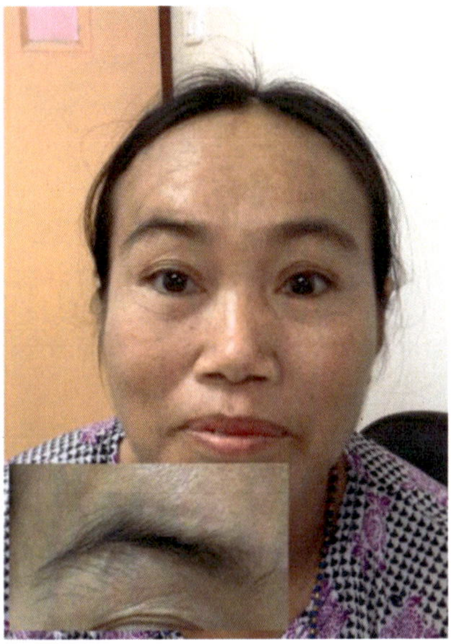

Figure 22. Skin appearance (6 months after the operation).

Skin Closure

In the beginning of KSA, cosmesis prevented many neurosurgeons from attempting this approach and led to the abandonment of KSA. Other than the incision making and the bone opening, skin closure is a very important step. All active bleeding points must be secured before skin suture. Layer-by-layer closure should be done, first by restoring the pericranial flap and the orbicularis oculi with absorbable sutures. Followed by the dermis closure using small size absorbable sutures with buried knots. The skin is approximated by 5-0 or 6-0 prolene intracutaneous method. Steri-Strips™ are then applied to the suture line for better cosmetic result. No drains are used in all cases. The excellent cosmetic result and patients' satisfaction can be expected if special care is properly taken (Figure 22).

Special Postoperative Care

The wound should be compressed by applying pressure using palms for 5-10 minutes to avoid hypodermal or subcutaneous hematoma. Then a cold pack should be applied with slight pressure over the incision for 24 hours. Failure to do this will increase the likelihood of postoperative hypodermal effusion and periorbital swelling resulting by blood leakage from loose tissues. Before applying the cold pack, some waterproof material should be applied over the Steri-Strips™ to prevent the wound from the contamination. The patient was observed overnight in the neurosurgical intensive care unit and then can be transferred to the ordinary ward. If no other unexpected complications occurred, then the patient can be discharged within a few days after the operation.

Limitations of KSA

Even though KSA has been used to access many lesions in the anterior skull base, it may not be appropriate for all lesions. Its limitation comes from the small opening of the skin and the craniotomy size. The narrow viewing angle through this small opening decreases the amount of light for adequate visualization of the deep-seated lesion. In order to compensate for this limitation, neurosurgeons are forced to adjust the microscope angle and sometimes the operating table more frequent. By adjusting those, visualization of the operative field will be better. However, after the era of the modern endoscope, neurosurgeons can also compensate for this limitation with the use of an endoscope. Another limitation related to the small opening is the inconvenient of the application of the microinstruments during the operation such as dissection, cutting, suction, and clipping. Routine bayonet-shaped microinstruments cannot be used conveniently through this small hole (Figure 23). Fortunately, new microinstruments with a coaxial shaft alleviate this problem (Figure 24). However, even though there are many innovative techniques and microinstruments, the most dreadful situation still persists. Vascular control for highly vascular lesions through the keyhole windows is quite difficult. To alleviate this problem, case selection is a very important factor during preoperative management [14].

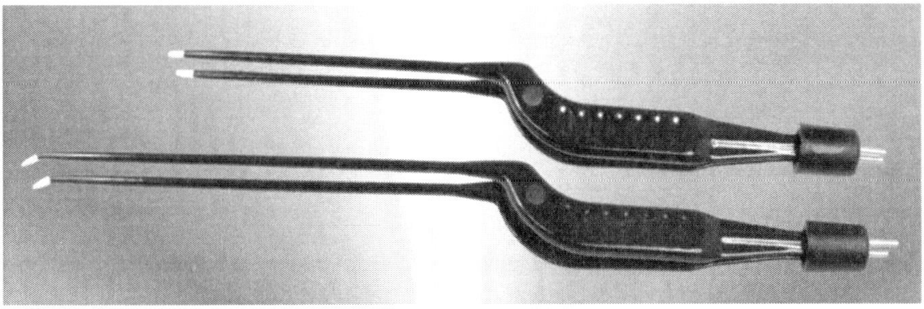

Figure 23. Ordinary bayonet-shaped microinstruments.

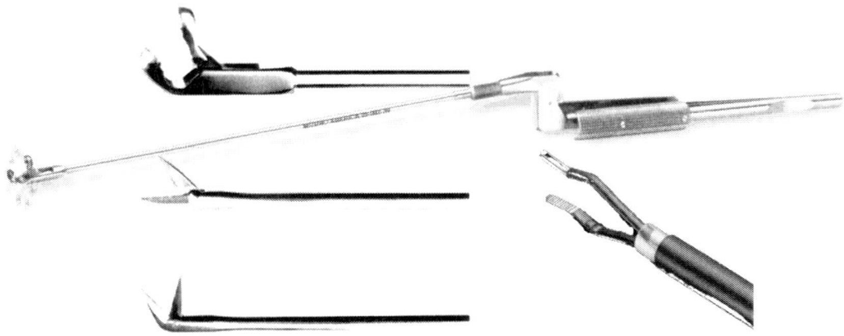

Figure 24. Coaxial shaft (slimmed) microinstruments.

Since KSA uses small incision with limited craniotomy size, this approach is appropriate for pituitary adenomas with or without suprasellar extension (Figure 25 A). However, in case of invasive adenomas that invade outside the sellar into parasellar area (extreme parasellar extension) (Figure 25 B), this approach is not suitable.

Another important disadvantage of KSA is its limitation in diminishing the opportunity for a change of plan if any unexpected events occur during the surgery. This resulted from its limited size for the surgical corridor. So case selection and preoperative planning is a very crucial step in every case.

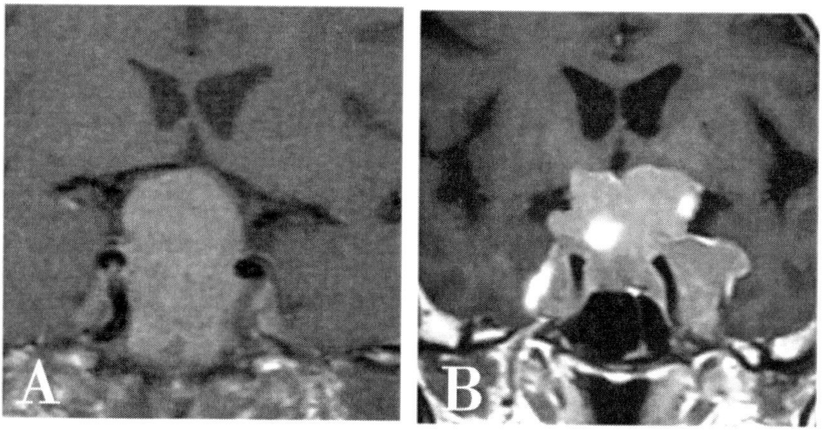

Figure 25. Pituitary adenoma with suprasellar extension (A) and invasive parasellar extension (B).

Complications Related to KSA

Complications found following KSA usually resulted from the limitation of the incision and the craniotomy size. Technically, we can classify the complications as follows.

Complications Related to Skin Incision

The most common complication found during this step is the supraorbital nerve injury. To avoid this complication, the incision must be limited lateral to the supraorbital notch/foramen. However, in some specific cases, extension of the incision lateral to this notch/foramen is unavoidable. Luckily, in such a case, this nerve usually recovers spontaneously within a few months.

Complication Related to the Frontal Sinus

Every attempt should be made to avoid opening the frontal sinus during craniotomy but in a large sinus, breakage into the sinus is possible. In such case, the frontal sinus should be separated from the operative field using betadine-soaked cottonoids during the whole operation. When the operation is finished, in order to avoid postoperative mucocele (Figure 26), there are 2 common procedures to deal with the frontal sinus. First by sinus obliteration, the sinus should be cleaned by removal of the sinus mucosal and packed with abdominal fat or muscle. Second, the sinus is cranialized by drilling out the inner table of the frontal sinus. All of the mucosa is stripped off and the frontonasal duct is obliterated (Figure 27). Failure to use enough precaution with the frontal sinus may cause postoperative mucocele or postoperative CNS infection.

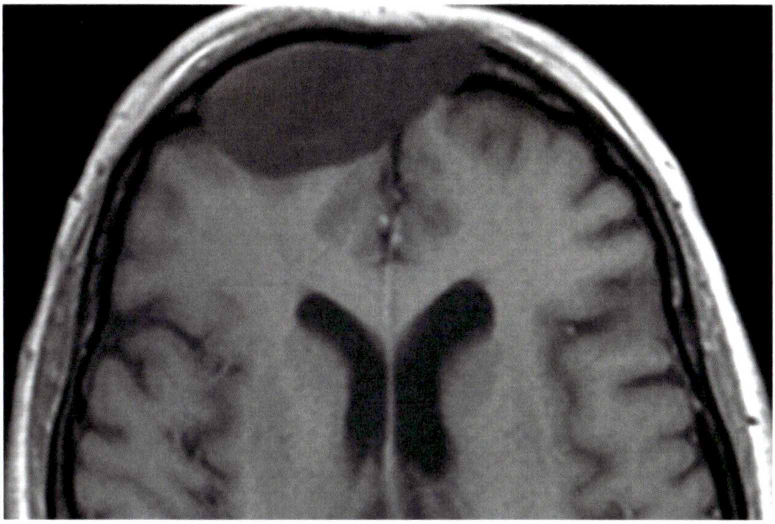

Figure 26. Frontal sinus mucocele.

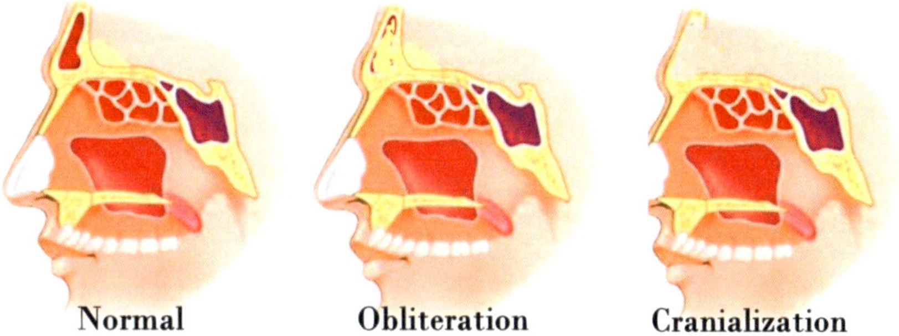

Figure 27. Two common procedures in handling frontal sinus. Obliteration by fat packing and cranialization by removal of inner table.

Complication Related to Craniotomy Size

This may be the most dangerous complication, if fatal bleeding from the internal carotid artery occurs during the operation. Efforts to stop massive bleeding via a small and limited incision are not easy. The best method may to avoid this complication, which is related to case selection and preoperative planning. Slim or coaxial microinstruments are very helpful in this situation. However, this limitation should not be overstated. Despite the small size of the craniotomy, slow CSF release proved to be large enough for safe surgical interventions without over retraction of the brain.

Complication Related to the Subfrontal Approach

Traction injury from the brain retractor can be avoided by releasing the CSF and applying more force to the frontal lobe via the subfrontal approach.

Complications Related to the Dural Closure

Every effort must be utilized to gain a watertight dural closure. Failure to do this will result in CSF leakage and meningitis.

KSA and Worldwide Opinions

Many different approaches for handling pituitary adenomas have been proposed. Among them, the most well-known one is "Pterional transsylvian approach." Even though this approach gives us wide exposure and wide scope of the surgical field; unnecessary exposure of the cortical area increases the risk of postoperative iatrogenic complications not directly associated with the lesion itself. After the minimally invasive concept has been implemented and accepted as a standard procedure in neurosurgery, numerous neurosurgeons started to develop their skills to serve many patients worldwide. The final clinical results of minimally invasive neurosurgery is remarkable and gives patients a shorter hospital stay and less morbidity.

KSA was popularized worldwide by many institutes because of its many advantages, especially the less traumatic and direct surgery that targeted the lesion within short distance. Many medical industries have innovated new microsurgical instruments to alleviate the limitation of keyhole surgery. With this approach, pituitary adenoma can be removed through a small opening about the size of a dime, visualizing the vital structures using a microscope.

There are numerous reports given to us about the pros and cons of KSA. Wiedemayer et al. reported an evaluation of KSA and its indications, advantages, and limitations [15]. They concluded that KSA was safe, effective, and time-sparing. Ormond et al. reviewed the evolution of KSA and stressed that KSA played a legitimate role in the armamentarium of the modern skull base surgeon, offering a less invasive but still efficacious approach to a number of lesions along the subfrontal corridor [16]. For newcomers who do not have enough experience and need more practical experience, a smaller, simpler lesion should be performed first before moving on to larger, more complicated ones. They suggested that midline and suprasellar lesions were more easily accessed through this approach than laterally-based lesions. From a study reported by Fatemi et al., both EETA and KSA can be used for non-pituitary adenoma patients such as craniopharyngioma and meningioma patients [17]. They found that the EETA was preferred for removal of most retrochiasmal craniopharyngiomas, whereas the supraorbital route was recommended for meningioma larger than 30 to 35 mm or with growth beyond the supraclinoid carotid arteries. For smaller midline tumors, either approach could be used, depending on the surgeon's experience and tumor anatomy.

From a cadaveric study that compared KSA and the traditional pterional approach reported by A. Perneczky, the difference in the area of exposure between both approaches was less than 1 cm, and there was no difference in the total or contralateral side area of exposure in the parasellar region [18]. He concluded that the limitations of KSA have more to do with "surgical freedom" of microinstruments than in the field of view at depth. Zhang Mao-shi et al. concluded in the Chinese Medical Journal that KSA offers many advantages: (1) Haircuts are not needed, thus decreasing the psychological burden affecting the patients, especially female patients. (2) A short skin incision, a simple and swift craniotomy, and limited (but sufficient) cerebral exposure are all beneficial to quick healing of wounds, to reducing approach-related morbidity, and to achieving shorter hospital stays. The length of the surgical procedure is significantly reduced as compared with standard techniques. (3) Although the exposures are small and limited, lesions can be accessed satisfactorily and removed smoothly. (4) The nerve and vascular supply to the temporal and frontal muscles are preserved. The short skin incision is hidden in the eyebrow, producing excellent cosmetic results. Patients can apply a tattoo to cover the eyebrow incision if necessary. They also concluded that KSA could be applied for numerous lesions in anterior cranial fossa surgery, such as anterior communicating artery aneurysm, olfactory groove meningioma, craniopharyngioma, planum sphenoidale meningioma, tuberculum meningioma, or parasellar lesion. In the final chapter of their report, they summarized that KSA offers almost equally effective surgical management to that of the conventional approaches, but results in less surgery-related morbidity. Thus, KSA is worthy of wide use. However, they also mentioned that KSA is not entirely suitable for large invasive pituitary adenomas and this approach should be performed by highly experienced neurosurgeons under well-equipped conditions.

EETA has many advantages when compared with KSA, such as no brain retraction, no visible scar, and less postoperative pain. But EETA has a higher risk of postoperative CSF leakage, especially after the extensive EETA for complex skull base tumors. While KSA may have some visible postoperative scars, the chance of postoperative CSF leakage is very low. If we combine the risk of postoperative CSF leakage together with the pros and cons of both approaches, KSA can be named as a "mini-invasive" approach [20].

It was already mentioned that keyhole via an eyebrow incision was applied in intracranial aneurysmal surgery, especially anterior circulation aneurysms. A paper published by Heung SK et al. concluded that KSA provided adequate visualization and safe surgical manipulation of anterior circulation aneurysms. It improved postoperative results and resulted in shorter hospitalization times, as there was a reduction in the risk of complications, which included chewing discomfort, temporal muscle weakness, scarification, and cosmetic disturbances. Those mentioned advantages are true not only for anterior circulation aneurysmal surgery but can be applied to pituitary adenoma surgery as well. However, preoperative diagnostic imaging is a very important factor in successful keyhole aneurysmal surgery. Each individual patient should be evaluated for the possibility of proximal control, direction of the aneurysm, and application of the aneurysm clip [21].

Another cadaveric study by Rodrigo Ramos-Zúñiga et al. was published in Neurosurgery. It reported the modification of KSA into a trans-supraorbital fashion by resection of the orbital arch and drilling some segments of the orbital roof [22]. This trans-supraorbital approach provided the potential for access to the following aneurysm sites and related vascular structures. They concluded that this modified approach could allow a wider view of the optic chiasm and the main supratentorial arteries of the brain with the use of minimal brain retraction. The trans-supraorbital approach also affords the surgeon better illumination and better visualization in the deep planes, so this approach allows many possible choices of position of the surgical instruments to avoid obstruction of light during the procedure. They also pointed out that this approach can achieve minimal brain retraction in three ways 1) the angle of approach changes 45 degrees when the orbital roof is removed, allowing access to the ipsilateral optic nerve 2) dissection and cistern drainage is possible at all levels and, in the case of the sylvian fissure, is possible at the opercular and frontobasal level; and 3) the position of the patient's head, with the postural support of gravity, allows access to all of the natural spaces in this microsurgical corridor. They stressed that this technique is a clear example of the advantage of combining two current surgical concepts, namely, cranial base surgery, and minimally invasive neurosurgery. However, the comments from the reviewers are very valuable. Reviewers suggested that additional experience is necessary before the superiority of this approach in cerebral aneurysm can be demonstrated. Less experienced neurosurgeons should use this approach in a highly selective group of aneurysmal patients. "Less is not always more" was the best comment to warn neurosurgeons before adopting this technique as a standard approach in all aneurysmal cases.

The paper published in Pediatric Neurosurgery by El Shafei H.I. made conclusions about another modification of KSA into the mini fronto-orbito-zygomatic (MFOZ) approach via an eyebrow incision in treating pediatric pathologies including pituitary adenoma [23]. He believed that the MFOZ approach has the advantages of a small cosmetic eyebrow incision and the skull base trajectory, thus reducing brain retraction and achieving the desired exposure with a good outcome. This modified approach using an eyebrow incision in pediatric patients is safe, effective, and both suitable and convenient for treating lesions, especially at the sellar region.

Chapter V

Which Method is Better in Minimally Invasive Neurosurgery for Pituitary Adenoma: EETA or KSA?

After the beginning of the endoscopic era, EETA was considered a true minimally invasive pituitary neurosurgery. Pituitary tumors could be removed without a visible surgical scar through the natural opening of the body (nostrils). Patients could be discharged within a few days after surgeries and could resume their normal activity within a week. Many reports confirmed that EETA was the true minimally invasive procedure and EETA was considered a first choice for pituitary adenoma surgery. However, EETA was not a surgery without complications. This approach still had some serious complications compared with the conventional pterional approach, especially the intraoperative bleeding incidence. Neurosurgeons had to stop arterial bleeding from the internal carotid artery through the deep and narrow space of the nostrils. This complication could be handled more easily under the pterional approach compared with EETA.

At the same time as EETA was developing, KSA was also popularized by many neurosurgeons. Since Donald H. Wilson first described the term "keyhole surgery" as an extension of limited trephinations. However, the aim of keyhole surgery is not only limited craniotomy but also limited brain exploration and minimal brain retraction. In short, the criteria of the keyhole concept is minimum iatrogenic neurotrauma but maximum efficiency in handling the lesions. The advantages may contribute to improved postoperative outcome including a shorter hospitalization time with fewer complications compared with conventional techniques. In case of a pituitary tumor and other suprasellar lesions, KSA is done using a small incision above and close to the eyebrow about 2-4 cm in length. This incision is placed just above the supraorbital prominence of the orbital wall. A small craniotomy with a diameter of only about 3-5 cm can be used as a door to attack most lesions in the skull base of the anterior cranial fossa. All of the critical neurovascular structures can be identified and handled through this small keyhole in the same way as a conventional one can be done. Many neurosurgeons claimed that this keyhole approach could be used instead of EETA. Surgeons can manipulate the above-mentioned vital structures more effectively and safer than the endonasal approach. Moreover, in case of an encased optic nerve and anterior circle of Willis, KSA seemed to be superior in terms of safe total removal than in EETA. For the above-mentioned reasons, some neurosurgeons claim that KSA may be safer than EETA for complex pituitary adenoma surgery. So it is very difficult to answer the question "Which is the better method in minimally invasive neurosurgery for pituitary adenoma?" If neurosurgeons wanted to perform both minimally invasive and safer surgery at the same time, they have to choose the most appropriate approach depending on the individual patient. Good knowledge of both approaches, familiarity of the surgeon, and the main drawback of each approach can guide the surgeon to the correct answer for the sake of the patient.

Pros and Cons between EETA vs. KSA

The minimally invasive concept is widely accepted as a first choice for many surgical procedures. For neurosurgery, since the modern counter-balanced mobile operating microscope was developed, the previous standard approach for pituitary adenoma surgery shifted from a large pterional craniotomy to other choices. In the beginning of minimally invasive surgery for pituitary adenoma, there were two common approaches: microscopic transseptal transsphenoidal and small pterional approach. But when the endoscopic era emerged and the high technology microscope was developed, EETA and KSA stepped over and were adopted as real minimally invasive surgery. As compared with EETA, KSA seems to be more invasive. But in the case of complex skull base tumors, there is a greater chance that the tumors will not be completely removed, especially in the lateral margin. In such a case, KSA is likely to be more seductive and can be named as a "mini-invasive" approach. However, both approaches have their own drawbacks.

Wongsirisuwan M summarized the pros and cons between EETA and KSA in many varieties [24].

Advantage of EETA

No Visible Scar

This may be the most outstanding advantage of EETA compared with other approaches. Using the endonasal space as the entrance to the sellar area means that there is no skin incision at all. In an easy case, without using a nasal speculum and no destruction of turbinate or nasal mucosa, the first anatomy that will be destroyed is the sphenoid ostium and the sphenoidal floor. However, the minimally invasive approach does not mean the operation will not leave a scar. Neurosurgeons have to be concerned with many factors before making the decision of choosing the best approach.

Recovery Period and Days of Admission

In most cases of EETA, the patients will have short recovery period and hospital stay. If they do not have any endocrinological problem, they can be discharged early. No need to return for taking stitches out.

Disadvantage of EETA

Transsphenoidal surgery, either microscopic or endoscopic, is considered a safe procedure for pituitary tumor removal, especially by experienced surgeons. However, this surgery may not a safe procedure so many factors could influence the success of this kind of operation.

Anatomical Variation of Endonasal Pathway

Although the endonasal pathway is a straight-forward route from the start of the opening of the nose up to the ostium of the sphenoid sinus, anatomical variations do occur frequently. This makes the surgery more difficult and requires a strong surgical knowledge of the endonasal anatomy. After the study of Sazgar et al., 63% of patients had septum deviations [25]. Concha bullosa presented up to 53% of patients and is often associated with the deviation of the nasal septum to the contralateral side [26]. This causes narrowing of the nasal lumen that can obscure the operative view, including the view during the introduction of surgical instruments. Another study that discovered septal deviation was performed by

Erik J van Lindert who described that 48% of patients have anatomical variations of endonasal pathway septum deviation [27]. Complications during EETA in the endonasal phase occurred in 3.8%. Confronting the anatomic variation of noses may be difficult for neurosurgeons. In such a case, an ear, nose and throat (ENT) surgeon could help neurosurgeons by operating in collaboration. EETA in case of an extremely narrowed nasal pathway can endanger the patient if there are bleeding problems during the operation, especially if the bleeding sources are from major arteries such as sphenopalatine or an internal carotid artery. A coordinated team effort with different specialists is advised to lessen this morbidity.

Image Guidance Needed

Imaged guidance is very important for the newcomers performing EETA. Although there are many useful landmarks during the endonasal approach, such as the nasal septum, middle turbinate, sphenoid ostium, and vomer plate, these landmarks also have many variations and cannot be easily recognized in some difficult cases. Using the C-arm fluoroscope or navigator is very helpful in such cases. This image guidance can help the surgeon when he encounters the anatomical disorientation during dissection. If he gets lost during the approach, a serious devastating situation can occur. For example, if the approach is out of the midline in the sphenoidal phase then the internal carotid artery can be injured and this complication could be fatal. Even directly approaching the midline, the anatomical variation of the internal carotid artery can still get in the way. To reduce the risk of deviation in preoperative evaluation in the nasal approach, either an MRI or CT scan is very important especially when neurosurgeons are in the learning curve period.

Mononostril vs. Binostril Approach

The nasal phase approach of EETA has two concepts. One preferred a mononostril while another advocated the binostril approach. The mononostril will harm nasal mucosa more than the binostril because surgeons need to put many instruments through only one passage. This can also make the surgery more difficult and may increase the degree of complications especially in the narrowed nasal passage of some races. In such cases, the patient may have breathing problems for the rest of their lives. To increase the space for the mononostril approach, surgeons often require removal of the middle turbinate. However, can this be considered as "minimally invasive"?

Skull Base Destruction and CSF Leakage

One of the major and serious complications of transsphenoidal approach (both conventional and endonasal) was cerebrospinal fluid (CSF) leakage. This complication was reported in many literatures and was known as a possible fatal complication. Especially in the hands of a less experienced surgeon, this complication could be more frequent. This complication was rarely seen in the conventional pterional approach and even in the supraorbital keyhole approach. The CSF leak was treated with external lumbar drainage or even reoperation, securing with a fat graft or dural repair (which is not easy). Another pitfall during the surgery, the Onodi cell (Sphenoethmoidal cell) may be mistaken for the sphenoid sinus (Figure 28). Removal of Onodi cell may lead to CSF leakage. This complication also seemed to occur less often with an experienced surgeon.

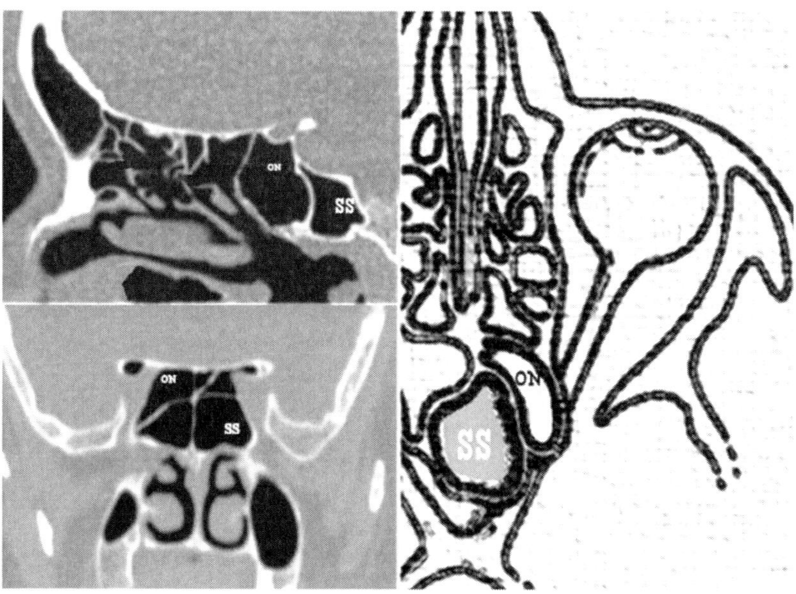

Figure 28. Onodi cell(ON) or Sphenoethmoidal recess (SS=Sphenoid Sinus).

Bleeding Control

Controlling the bleeding in any deep and narrowed space is a nightmare for neurosurgeons. This complication strictly relates to the approach. In pituitary tumor surgery, neurosurgeons are more familiar with controlling bleeding through the pterional approach much more than the transsphenoidal approach. Even if the bleeding could be controlled successfully, patients might have a severe epistaxis later. The sphenopalatine artery at the inferolateral border of the middle turbinate was one of the most common bleeding sources and must be completely secured during the operation. Some patients result in shock from sphenopalatine artery bleeding. Another major source of bleeding was from the internal carotid artery, especially if there was an anatomical disorientation with loss of route, which occurred during the sphenoidal phase. Uncontrolled bleeding can force the neurosurgeons to abort the procedure and shift to conventional surgery. To lessen this, image guidance can restore the anatomical disorientation.

Suprasellar Manipulation

Most cases of pituitary tumor have suprasellar and parasellar extensions. In such cases, the patients will complain of a visual problem. Even though transsphenoidal surgery can remove an intrasellar tumor clearly, removing the suprasellar part is not easy because of the higher extension of the suprasellar part and the deeper surgical depth. Some cases of pituitary tumors have adhesion with the surrounding structures; clearing the tumor from these structures using an endoscope is not easy at all. There are many limitations using the endoscope in the deep space of EETA compared with microscope. One of them is a one or two-handed surgery, which will be discussed next.

Advantage of Keyhole Supraorbital Approach (KSA)

Familiarity of Surgeon

The basic KSA is much like the subfrontal approach combined with the pterional approach. Surgeons can operate in a familiar way. Most of the critical landmarks can be visualized under the microscope. The new innovated magnetic and counter-balanced microscope makes the surgeon more comfortable in such a long operative time compared with the endoscopic procedure. Moreover, craniotomy skill is much easier compared with the endoscopic skill in view of most neurosurgeons. Under critical situations, familiarity with the approach may save the life of the patients.

Simple Instruments

Compared with EETA, the basic craniotomy set is much simpler than the endoscopic set. Patients undergoing KSA need no image guidance. On the contrary, keyhole surgery needs simple anatomical landmarks such as olfactory tract, internal carotid artery, optic nerve and chiasm, pituitary stalk, and planum sphenoidale, which can be visualized under direct vision or microscopic view. These landmarks allow the surgeons to follow their path easier than EETA. With

EETA, this approach needs a new separate set of instruments. Most of them are expensive and can be used only in specific surgical operations. In a hospital where cost-benefit is a great concern, keyhole craniotomy is the best solution.

Microscopic vs. Endoscopic Skill of Surgeon

Skilled handling of the endoscope is new and demands more surgical experience for newcomers. Microscope visualization is in three dimensions whereas the endoscope is only in two dimensions. Under 3D, a neurosurgeon can utilize his surgical skill during pituitary tumor surgery better than in 2D. Endoscopic endosinus surgery is relatively new to neurosurgeons; this makes many neurosurgeons lack endoscopic skills, which may cause fatal complications in critical situations, especially when confronting them together with anatomical variations. However, for ENT surgeons, they are already well-experienced with the endoscopic sinus approach. For this reason, some neurosurgeons prefer to perform EETA in collaboration with an ENT surgeon.

Variety of Applications

Appropriate case selection for EETA is one of the gold measures in successful surgery. To remove the tumor under a deep and narrow space like the EETA, the tumor should be easily suckable. In some pituitary tumors, the tumor itself is not easily sucked. Neurosurgeons need bipolar cauterization and a sharp cut with specially designed microscissors, this procedure may traumatize critical structures such as the internal carotid artery or hypophyseal branch of the pituitary gland. Sometimes, neurosurgeons planned to remove an easily suckable pituitary tumor using EETA but finally found that the tumor could not be easily sucked. If they continue operation under this situation, the operative time must be extended and this increases the risk of complications afterwards. In the case of KSA, almost all of the lesions in the sellar and suprasellar area can be removed using KSA. These lesions are not only pituitary tumors but also include non-pituitary tumors such as craniopharyngioma, meningioma, and vascular lesion.

Bilateral Free Hands

Operations done under bilateral free hands is much more comfortable for the neurosurgeon, especially in critical situations. For example, bleeding control from the main arterial source is very difficult to stop with only one free hand, like in EETA. Even though neurosurgeons use self-endoscopic holding devices, bleeding control under bilateral free hands is still not a piece of cake. The lens surface of the endoscope will be obscured by the blood stream. Under KSA, surgeons will have bilateral free hands at all times. This makes neurosurgeons feel more comfortable during the whole period in the operating theatre.

Removing Encased Tumors

In a large pituitary tumor with massive suprasellar or parasellar extension, the tumor has a great likelihood to encase the vital structures such as arteries of the Circle of Willis, optic nerve, optic chiasm, or optic tract. Under EETA, it is impossible to remove this encased tumor. Surgeons can only decompress these nearby structures. However, under KSA, removing this encased lesion is much easier and safer. Using a microscope, with or without an endoscope-assisted technique, either decompression or removal of these encased tumors is easier, compared with EETA.

Bleeding Control

Most cases of pituitary tumors can control bleeding easily using cottonoid together with surgical packing. Other bleeding control materials such as gel foam, Helitene®, Avitene® are also helpful. However, if the bleeding point is from a main arterial bleed, like hypophyseal artery or the more serious source like the internal carotid artery, bleeding control in such a deep and narrow space like EETA may be an apocalypse. Under KSA, bleeding control is much easier, even from major sources as mentioned above.

CSF Leakage

Under EETA, surgeons have to reconstruct the sellar floor and sphenoid sinus carefully. If CSF comes out of this channel, lumbar drainage or reoperation is mandated. However, in the KSA group, surgeons can repair the dura in a watertight fashion. In case of dural shortening, fascia combined with Bioglue® is very helpful.

Recovery Time and Days of Admission

Compared with EETA, patients operated under KSA have a rapid recovery time. Most patients can be extubated immediately after the operation. In cases without endocrine problems, they can be discharged within a few days. This is the same as in the EETA group.

Disadvantage of KSA

Special Designed Instruments

As described by Perneczky, if the craniotomy is smaller than 15 mm then the intraoperative use of conventional microinstruments becomes very limited. Development of new tube-shaft microinstruments is mandatory for performing keyhole surgery. These specially designed microinstruments are very expensive compared with conventional microinstruments in the basic microneurosurgical set.

Visible Scar

The distinct difference between EETA and KSA seems to be the visible scar of KSA. EETA uses the nasal pathway as the door to the sellar region while KSA uses the supraorbital area, so KSA leaves the visible scar just next to the eyebrow. To hide this scar, meticulous subcuticular suture can alleviate this problem. In case of serious concern, collaboration with a plastic surgeon may be helpful. However, most scars will fade out after 3-4 months and are hardly seen after 6-12 months (Figure 29). In clinical practice, most patients do not care about the visible scar as much as the result and the safety of the operation using KSA. For EETA, there will be no visible scar at all. However, in some cases, operations will leave a nasal anomaly such as septal deviation resulting in breathing difficulty. Though this deviation is not visible, it makes the patients uncomfortable for the rest of their life.

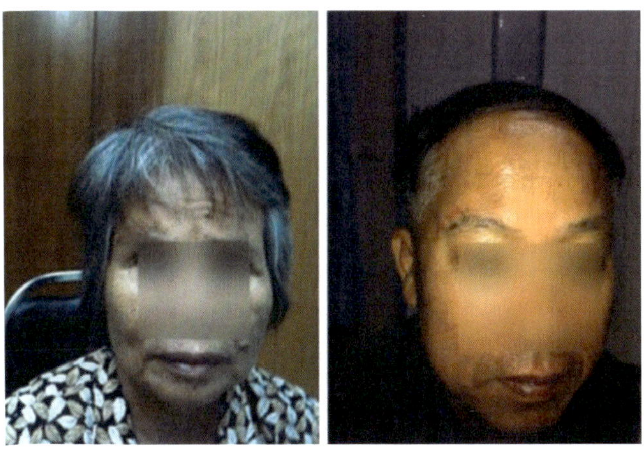

Figure 29. Visible scar: 2 weeks after keyhole supraorbital surgery. However, scar will be hardly seen after 6 months.

Another visible scar is from the craniotomy border. To perform the craniotomy, the surgeon must make an initial burr hole first. Cutting the skull using a craniotome, there will be a skull defect that can be seen through the forehead. Using the small diameter blade of craniotome and making a small initial hole using a small diameter drill are very helpful in hiding this visible scar. Using Flapfix®, Craniofix®, or a Titanium miniplate is very helpful to hide the burr defect. Bone filling substitute can also be used to hide the craniotomy defect.

Numbness of Forehead and Facial Asymmetry

To enter the supraorbital margin, the incision must cut through the supraorbital nerve. This will leave numbness above the incision area and make the wrinkle of the ipsilateral side disappear. This facial asymmetry can be seen clearly, when the patients express facial appearance. Like the visible scar problem, most cases will have spontaneous recovery within 6-12 months. In some selected cases, surgeons can avoid this complication by making an incision lateral to the supraorbital nerve.

Endocrine Problem

Entering the sellar and suprasellar area using KSA has a main difference when compared with the EETA in that the KSA will reach the suprasellar and pituitary stalk first, whereas the EETA will reach the sellar first and rarely reach up to the pituitary stalk. Mobilizing or injuring the stalk during KSA will aggravate postoperative diabetes insipidus. To alleviate this complication, surgeons must try to identify the stalk as early as possible before cutting or cauterizing the tumor.

Intrasellar View

This seems to be the major disadvantage of KSA. Since KSA enters the suprasellar and intrasellar region in the same way as the pterional approach, it will have a clear view of the suprasellar region but not for the intrasellar view. Under microscopic view from above (pterional or KSA), the intrasellar region is the blind spot. To reveal this blind spot, removal of the planum sphenoidale using a high-speed drill may be helpful. However, surgeons must use a great effort while drilling this area because there are lots of critical structures such as the optic nerve and arteries of anterior circulation. The endoscope-assisted microscopic approach is very helpful in this situation. The endoscope can pass through the keyhole gateway while surgeons can operate under the microscope at the same time. In many cases, the endoscope can also reveal not only the intrasellar area but also the undersurface of the optic nerves. Surgeons can achieve total tumor removal in this blind spot using both microscope and endoscope.

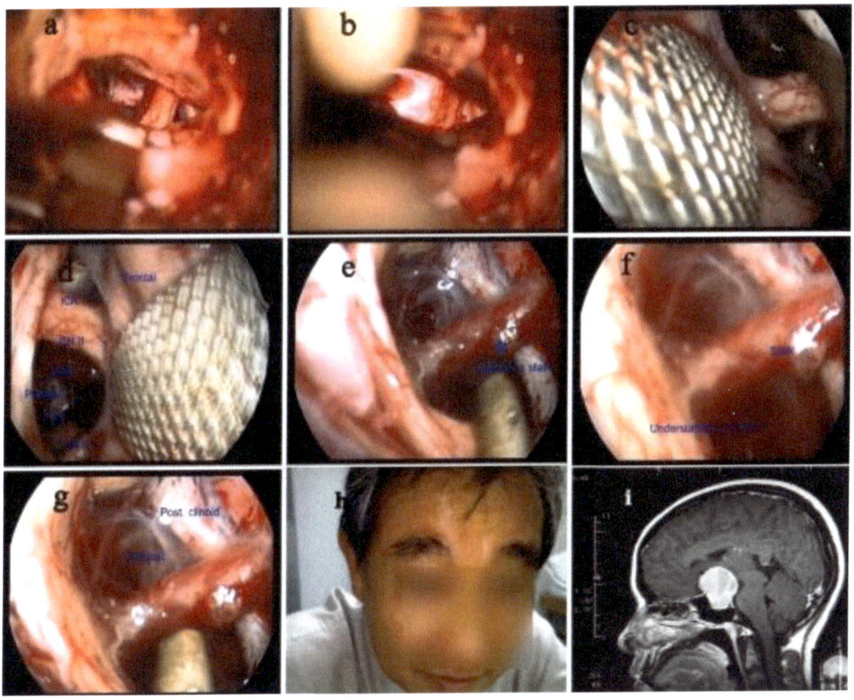

Figure 30. "Minimally invasive-maximally effective": Combination use of endoscope and microscope as "Endoscopic assisted microneurosurgery via KSA" of large sellar and suprasellar tumor. (a) view under microscope (after subtotal removal by microscope) (b) endoscope was passed through the keyhole (c) and (d) views under endoscope (e) asterisk (*) is the remaining tumor attached with the stalk (f) pituitary stalk and undersurface of optic chiasm (g) closer view of endoscope demonstrated remaining tumor, Lilequist's membrane and posterior clinoid process (h) patient 6 months after the operation (rarely visible scar) (i) Preoperative MRI.

In the final part of this report, he concluded that EETA has less approach-related morbidity in pituitary adenoma surgery. Other than conventional pterional approach or conventional transsphenoidal approach, neurosurgeons can use this approach as an armamentarium in handling a pituitary tumor. EETA is truly a minimally invasive procedure in removing the pituitary tumor. However, truly minimal invasive surgery does not mean only the operation without a scar or operation with short recovery period. It should have enough safety for the patients themselves. Some serious complications are approach-related complications such as a bleeding problem or CSF leakage. In a very difficult EETA case, having KSA in armamentarium as a minimally invasive procedure may help surgeons avoid unnecessary complications. To achieve a good outcome under a minimally invasive concept, neurosurgeons must select the most appropriate approach based upon his experience and skill.

The answer to the question "Which is the better choice in minimally invasive neurosurgery for pituitary adenoma?" is not an easy one. In some situations, KSA may be superior than EETA and vice versa. EETA may be superior to KSA in the view of "less approach-related" morbidity whilst KSA is superior to EETA in the view of a "more versatile" approach. However, truly minimal invasive surgery does not mean only the operation without a scar or operation with a short recovery period. It should provide enough safety for the patients themselves. Some serious complications are approach-related complications such as a bleeding problem or CSF leakage. In a very difficult EETA case, having KSA in armamentarium as a minimally invasive procedure may help surgeons avoid unnecessary complications. To achieve a good outcome under a minimally invasive concept, neurosurgeons must select the most appropriate approach based upon their experience and skill and they should follow the golden rule of thumb that is "minimally invasive-maximally effective" (Figure 30).

Chapter VI

Radiation Therapy and Pituitary Adenomas

KSA and EETA are not the only minimally invasive techniques for handling pituitary adenomas; radiation therapy is also categorized as a minimally invasive treatment. Radiation therapy uses high energy x-rays or particles to destroy tumor cells. The source of the radiation is from the machine base outside the patients' body. Usually, radiation therapy is reserved as an option when surgery is not possible. Every patient must know the pros and cons of what they are going to have by discussing with the surgeon and his team. Before radiation therapy starts, patients must be scanned (MRI) to calculate the exact size and boundary of the tumor. When all data are obtained then the appropriate dose and shape of the radiation beams is prepared.

Conventional Radiation

Conventional radiation therapy is the most common type of radiotherapy for cancer treatment. It attacks the cancerous cells by blocking their growth ability. Usually, the proper dose will be divided into smaller fractions and each fraction will be delivered per day during the entire course, which may last 5 days a week for one or two months. The ionizing radiation will damage the cancerous DNA leading to cellular death. So, it is imperative to prevent the surrounding healthy tissues from this ionizing radiation. The use of conventional radiotherapy in non-malignant conditions is worrisome because of the risk of the radiation-induced cancer. In pituitary adenomas, conventional therapy is usually followed by hypopituitarism because it is impossible to control the target area by conventional radiotherapy.

Stereotactic Radiation

Stereotactic radiation is a modified external beam radiation therapy. For conventional external beam radiation (2DXRT), the machine will deliver the radiation using two-dimensional beams, whereas stereotactic radiation will deliver three-dimensional beams. The main drawback of 2DXRT is that some high-dose treatments may be limited by the radiation toxicity capacity of the surrounding healthy tissues, which are in close contact to the target area. For pituitary adenomas the optic apparatus, which is usually close to the adenoma, is very sensitive to radiation. So, 3DXRT, like stereotactic radiation, will be more suitable for many brain tumors.

Stereotactic radiation has many advantages over conventional radiation because it can deliver the right amount of radiation in a short time and its accuracy is very high. So, we can call stereotactic radiation, radiosurgery (surgery without knife), because it does not use a blade to destroy the tumor cell. We can classify radiosurgery into three basic forms according to technological equipment and source of radiation.

(1) Gamma knife® (using Cobalt-60 gamma radiation)
(2) LINAC (Photon therapy)
(3) Proton beam therapy (using heavy charged particles-protons)

Among them, the cobalt-60 based machine is widely used for brain lesions. This machine provides extremely accurate targeting and precise treatment. When combined with the stereotactic frame, it provides excellent results for many types of intracranial lesions, and is known as "Gamma Knife®." It creates less damage to normal healthy brain tissue but unfortunately; it can only be used for some small lesions (less than 3-4 cm). While LINAC is capable of treating larger volume lesions using multiple consecutive sessions called "fractionated radiosurgery." The well-known LINACs are Novalis® and Cyberknife®. This system is superior to Gamma knife® because it can be used not only in the brain but also for the whole body. However Gamma knife® is superior to LINAC because LINAC must move during the treatment so its accuracy is less than Gamma knife®.

As previously mentioned, radiosurgery is surgery using radiation. It destroys the selected lesion precisely by ionizing radiation rather than excision with a surgical blade. The most well-known radiosurgery is credited to that created by the Swedish neurosurgeon, "Lars Leksell," as a single high dose fraction of radiation. However, this technology must work in collaboration with good medical imaging to target the lesion precisely. He combined the radiosurgery together with the three-dimensional coordinate system named "Stereotactic Radiosurgery, SRS." These combined systems enable the accurate correlation of a virtual target obtained by image guidance, and were used to destroy the targeted lesion. SRS was first used to destroy small lesions in the brain that were amenable to conventional surgery (surgery with knife) by crossfiring the intracranial target from multiple directions with narrow beams of radiation. The beam paths converge in the target volume, delivering a lethal cumulative dose of radiation, while limiting the dose in the adjacent healthy tissue. This concept made SRS compatible with intracranial lesions because the healthy intracranial tissues surrounding the lesions are very important and must be preserved at all cost.

For a time, SRS was significantly developed; it has been widely used in many areas of the body. Many models have been created, such as Gamma knife®, LINAC (Linear Particle Accelerator), and Cyberknife®. However, significant clinical judgment must be used with this equipment, and considerations must include lesion type, pathology if available, size, location, age, and general health of the patient. Radiosurgery outcome may not be evident for months or years after the treatment. Radiosurgery does not remove any tumors, but results in a biological inactivation of the tumor (tumor control), lack of growth of the lesion is normally considered treatment success.

Proton Beam Therapy (Figure 31)

Proton beam therapy is a type of radiotherapy but it has some differences with conventional radiotherapy. Conventional therapy uses high-energy beams of radiation to destroy cancerous cells, but it creates serious damage to the surrounding tissues. This leads to many side effects such as hair loss, headache, nausea, vomiting, and can seriously affect the sensitive nervous system especially the visual apparatus system. Whereas, proton beam therapy uses the positive parts of atoms (proton) to kill the tumor cells. The killing effect of proton beam therapy comes from the accelerated protons that speed up by a particle accelerator and are then beamed into the target area. Another main different mechanism of proton beam therapy, as compared with conventional radiotherapy, is that it stops immediately once it hits the target cells so it results in much less damage to the normal nearby cells ("enter tissue, hit target, and stop"), whereas x-rays from conventional radiotherapy releases energy both before and after they hit the target area. So, the main chief advantage of proton beam therapy over conventional radiotherapy is that it can more precisely localize the radiation dose to the target area with less effect to the surrounding structures. The charged particles will destroy the DNA of cells, ultimately killing them or stopping their reproduction. The higher the rate of cell division, the more vulnerable the target cells. Hence, normal cells have a lower rate of cell division so it reduces damage to the surrounding tissue. After this principle, proton beam therapy is used most often to treat brain tumors in young children whose brains are still developing.

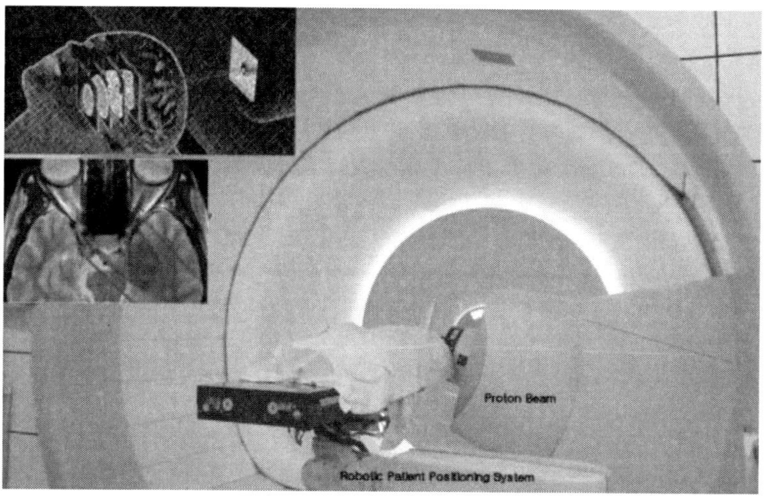

Figure 31. Proton beam therapy.

Proton beam therapy is usually recommended for irregularly shaped lesions that are located near critical structures. It has high potential to deliver high dose radiation in just minutes, directly within the boundaries of the tumors with minimal toxic effect to the nearby structures, so it is suitable for pituitary adenomas.

The main drawback of proton beam therapy is the availability of this equipment. Due to its complexity, it requires a highly specialized center with personnel to maintain safety. The cost-benefit is another main drawback due to its sophisticated technology.

Due to its availability, there are scant reports of using proton therapy in treating pituitary adenomas. In a study by Brian B. Ronson et al., they concluded that fractionated conformal proton-beam irradiation achieved effective radiologic, endocrinological, and symptomatic control of pituitary adenomas [28]. Significant morbidity was uncommon, with the exception of postradiation hypopituitarism. However, there is still a question about the effectiveness of proton beam therapy. It may cause less damage to healthy tissue but it is still unclear if it is good enough in destroying cancerous cells as the conventional radiotherapy.

However, proton beam therapy is a relatively new technology and just launched into the commercial market, so it demands a period of time and a greater number of cases to prove itself useful in treating pituitary adenomas.

Gamma Knife® (Figure 32)

Gamma knife® therapy is one of the most precise, powerful and proven treatments for many brain tumors. It delivers an invisible knife through the skin without a single cut or hair shaving to destroy the deep-seated tumor hiding under the skull. It contains multiple small cobalt-60 sources of gamma rays placed in a circular array in a heavily shielded assembly. A primary collimator aims the radiation emitted by these sources to a common focal point. The patient's head is held in place by a metal head frame called a "stereotactic frame" that is fixed to the skull by metallic pins. When the patient is brought into the station, his head will be firmly fixed with the machine so it can deliver a single, finely focused, high dose radiation to the target with little damage to surrounding tissue. The accuracy is less than 0.5 mm. The dose is typically prescribed at 50% to obtain the maximum dose at the focal point (center) and a minimal dose at the target edge.

There are many advantages to Gamma Knife® therapy:

- High precision: Its accuracy is less than 0.5 mm so the target is shot precisely under careful planning by a well-trained staff. The surrounding healthy tissue will be left intact and free from radiation.
- Patient friendly: It requires only one visit to complete its job. Patients usually need no admission. In brief, Gamma Knife® is a one-time therapy completed in a single day.

- High safety: It needs no general anesthesia so it is suitable for unhealthy patients with serious underlying risk factors. However, in some cases, light sedation may be needed to alleviate the scare and calm the patient.
- Painless treatment: Since it needs no surgical blade, there is no incision and no bleeding. The only possible pain comes from the fixation of the stereotactic frame but it should be handled by local anesthesia prior to pin fixation.
- Less radiation side effects: With careful planning, patients can tolerate Gamma Knife® surgery better than conventional radiotherapy. Acute radiation toxicity is very uncommon while late toxicity is very low. The safety from radiation of Gamma Knife® depends on the accuracy of target planning.

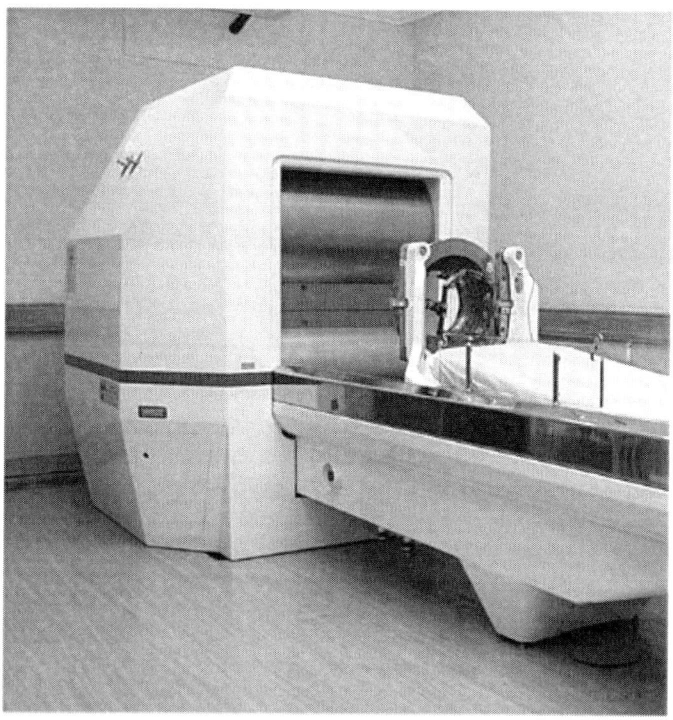

Figure 32. Gamma knife®.

However, there is no treatment without drawbacks. The main drawbacks of Gamma Knife® are:

- Size limitation: It is usually suitable for lesions less than 1 inch in diameter.
- Collaboration: During pin fixation of the stereotactic frame, the patient should collaborate with the doctor until the radiation is delivered to the target site. This step may be impeded in cases of young age groups.
- Induced hypopituitarism: This complication varies with the dose and accuracy in defining the target. Its risk increases during the period after radiosurgery.
- Optic nerve neuropathy: This seems to be the most serious complication after radiosurgery for treating pituitary adenoma. The risk increases if the target-nerve distance is less than 5 mm or the radiation dose is more than 8 Gy.

Since it is considered to be minimally invasive, Gamma Knife® radiosurgery has emerged as an important treatment modality for specific conditions of pituitary adenoma. There are numerous reports that supported the efficacy of Gamma Knife® in pituitary adenomas. In a study by Jason P Sheehan et al., they found that Gamma Knife surgery appears to be both safe and effective in treating nonfunctioning pituitary adenomas [29]. Long-term tumor control rates of 93% can be achieved in nonfunctioning pituitary adenomas. The risks of endocrinopathy, and visual dysfunction associated with radiosurgery appear to be quite low.

For functioning pituitary adenomas, Raef FA Hafez et al. reported that Gamma Knife® surgery is a safe and highly effective treatment for secretory pituitary adenoma patients who failed to achieve hormonal control after medical treatment alone, intolerant to its side effects, or post-operative with residual functioning adenoma or recurrence [30]. It is a safe and effective method for controlling secretory pituitary adenoma growth and inducing hormonal control, especially microadenoma with low morbidity, and could be a primary minimal invasive option.

After Gamma Knife® treatment, tumor control was observed for most pituitary adenomas and occurred gradually over a period of several years. A small increase in tumor size might be observed in the first 6 months after radiosurgery. In most cases, reductions in tumor size were not accompanied by a change in contrast enhancement or cyst formation [32].

For long-term results of Gamma Knife® radiosurgery for pituitary adenomas, it was effective and safe for the treatment of pituitary adenomas. However, the treatment strategies should be specific to each adenoma type according to the radiosensitivity, chemosensitivity and biological nature of the tumor. Nonfunctioning adenomas showed higher control rates than functioning adenomas even with lower dose treatment. Cushing disease showed the best response because of the smallest tumor size with the highest dose treatment. Acromegaly and prolactinoma were difficult to control because of larger tumors with lower dose treatment. The rate of hormone normalization was also high in Cushing disease but lower in prolactinoma and lowest in acromegaly. High-dose treatment was necessary for functioning adenomas to control tumor growth and over-secretion of hormones [32].

In brief, most of the studies concluded that Gamma Knife® offers a satisfactory risk-to-benefit ratio. It has generally favorable outcomes with low incidence of morbidity and essentially zero mortality. However, it should be proposed in cases of small target volume, sufficiently far from the optic apparatus to avoid the risk of radiation-induced optic neuropathy.

Linear Accelerator Based Radiotherapy (LINAC) (Figure 33)

There are some differences between LINAC and Gamma Knife® radio-surgery. Gamma Knife® uses gamma rays from the decay of Cobalt-60 while a LINAC produces X0rays from the impact of accelerated electrons striking a high z target. LINAC emits high energy x-rays or “photon” therapy while Gamma Knife® gets the gamma ray from the emitted radioisotope, which is usually cobalt-60.

Instead of using the Cobalt sources, LINAC emits high energy x-rays (photon therapy) from high voltage accelerators. Like the Gamma Knife®, patients under LINAC treatment will be immobilized in a fixed frame and treatment is delivered to the target area. The radiation dose of LINAC is more homogenous if compared with Gamma Knife®, so LINAC has an advantage in larger lesions as compared with Gamma Knife®. Using LINAC for brain lesions, the most suitable device should have 6 MeV of energy. It is capable of achieving extremely narrow beam geometries, such as 0.15 to 0.3 mm, therefore it can be used for multiple kinds of surgeries.

Like Gamma Knife, LINAC has also been used for treating pituitary adenomas. There were several reports worldwide using LINAC for pituitary adenomas. After Runge MJ et al., 61 nonsecreting pituitary adenomas were treated with a follow-up of more than 12 month [33]. They found that local tumor control was achieved up to 98% without any visual complications. They also concluded that LINAC is a minimally invasive, safe, and effective treatment for recurrent nonsecreting pituitary adenomas or microsurgically inaccessible residual tumors. It yielded a high rate of local long-term tumor control with a small number of radiation-induced side effects.

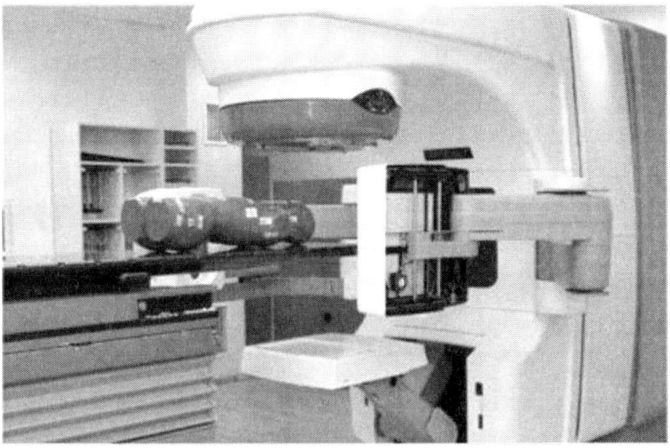

Figure 33. LINAC.

Another report that confirmed LINAC is a safe, effective treatment for pituitary adenomas belongs to Muramatsu J et al. [34]. They retrospectively evaluated the results of LINAC for pituitary adenoma. Tumor size decreased by less than 50% after LINAC treatment, with no recognizable regrowth of any of the tumors. In two out of four growth hormone-secreting adenomas, hormonal overproduction normalized, while the other two showed reduced hormonal production. One prolactin-secreting adenoma did not respond. Reduction of visual acuity and field was seen in one of thirteen patients. None of the patients developed brain radionecrosis or radiation-induced hypopituitarism.

Using LINAC as compared with conventional pituitary irradiation treatment was reported after presentation at the 38th annual meeting of the American society for Therapeutic Radiology and Oncology in 1996. Sei-Chul Yoon et al. tried to determine the impact of LINAC on the clinical course, hormonal status, and follow-up CT/MRI scan of pituitary macroadenomas [35]. After eight years of LINAC treatment in pituitary adenomas, 24 patients were treated. In all cases, they were surgically resected and followed by LINAC treatment. The mean follow-up period is 49.2 months and their results were compared to the results using conventional radiation. Overall, results revealed that LINAC could be used effectively in patients with pituitary adenoma. A more rapid hormonal and clinical response was achieved with LINAC than with conventional pituitary irradiation treatment.

Another interesting question regarding usage between Gamma Knife® and LINAC, is their clinical effectiveness and cost. In a study by Stefan Mathis et al., patients with primary brain tumors, brain metastases, arteriovenous malformations or trigeminal neuralgia were included in this study [36]. He found that Gamma Knife® is suitable for small lesions (better conformity, efficient workflow), while LINAC has advantages with bigger volumes (faster, better coverage, homogenity). From a cost perspective the LINAC system seem to be more versatile in its use, and is therefore recommended when radiosurgery case numbers are small. Local variables (consented indications, case numbers, existing equipment, experience of personnel) should be carefully evaluated to allow a decision that meets criteria of efficient patient care.

Cyberknife® (Figure 34)

LINAC has also been modified to treat more diseases. The most popular one is the frameless robotic "Cyberknife®." Cyberknife® does not use a frame to hold the patient, as a computer monitors the patient's position during treatment, using fluoroscopy. The computer allows tracking the tumor, rather than fixing the patient with a stereotactic frame. That's why it is called "frameless radiosurgery." Since no frame is needed, Cyberknife® can be extended to treat extracranial lesions such as spine lesions, prostatic tumors, lung cancers, and intraabdominal lesions. Cyberknife® can also be used for hypofractionated regimens in patients with tumors involving the optic apparatus that are not suitable for simple radiosurgery.

Cyberknife® has two main components working in collaboration:

(1) Radiation source: the radiation produced from a small linear particle accelerator.
(2) Robotic arm: this arm can move freely, which allows the energy to be directed at any part of the body from any direction.

In order to deliver the radiation precisely, Cyberknife® must use an accurate image guidance system. It will track the target lesion in real time during treatment. This imaging guidance allows Cyberknife® to deliver radiation with an accuracy of 0.5 mm without patients' immobilization. So, it is a kind of "frameless stereotactic radiosurgery." The image guidance system of Cyberknife® is a very sophisticated one. For intracranial lesions, the skull based tracking or the so-called "6D®" is used. 6D® are made for the 3 translational motions (X, Y and Z) with an additional 3 rotational motions. But for spinal lesions, the so-called "Xsight-spine®" is used instead. Since the spine can move relative to each other, the algorithms for the spine motion is more complicated in order to detect every motion of the spine during treatment.

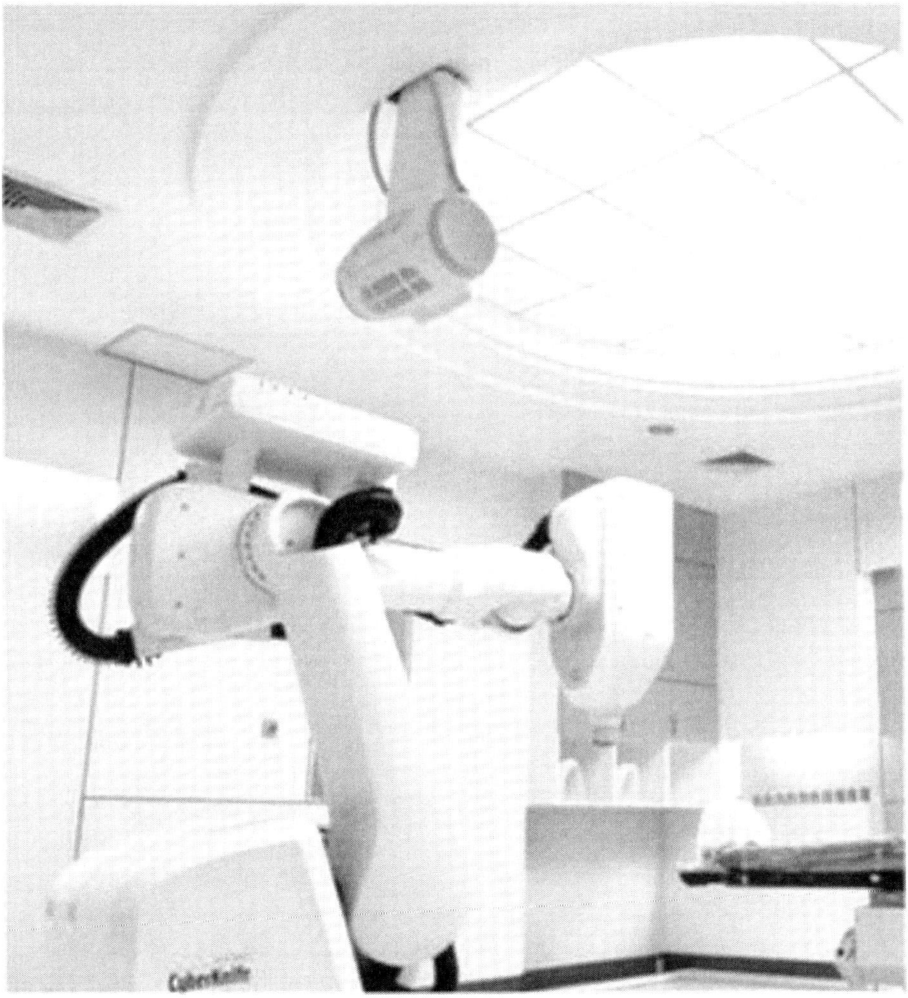

Figure 34. Cyberknife®.

When the Cyberknife® works in real clinical conditions, the radiation exposure to the surrounding healthy tissue is minimized as much as possible, but the level of the radiation exposure at the required target area is high enough to kill the cells of the targeted lesion. With its high accuracy, the dose of radiation can be raised to increase the likelihood of radiosurgical success. One common question is its accuracy, because it can be done without any frame or limitation of the patients' movement. The slow-dose X-ray camera is the key to this question. They can detect any movement that was created during the actual treatment; those movements will be signaled to the workstation in real time. The Cyberknife®'s computer-controlled robotic arm will compensate for any changes, even the breathing of the patient. When the patient breathes, the synchrony respiratory tracking system will sync with the station and the feedback will be compensated for high accuracy.

Another advantage of Cyberknife® technology is the advantage of multisession radiosurgery because it needs no stereotactic frame fixation. Patients can tolerate the Cyberknife® more than Gamma Knife®. The incidence of pituitary dysfunction (hypopituitarism) is much lower due to its multi-session radiosurgery.

As previously mentioned, Cyberknife® is frameless radiosurgery. It can be used for extracranial lesions including the spine. Benign or malignant tumors of the vertebra and spinal cord can be treated with Cyberknife® as well as the spinal arteriovenous malformation. In cases of spinal malignancies, Cyberknife® is very effective with pain control created by the tumor. For the non-spherical structure like the nerve, Cyberknife® can be used to treat trigeminal neuralgia.

With its sophisticated technology, Cyberknife® is also considered a non-invasive treatment for a wide range of lesions. It attacks hard-to-reach targets almost anywhere in the human body without incisions, anesthesia, or an overnight hospital stay. It is a pain-free surgery. Because of its precision, more powerful and effective doses of radiation can be administered as compared with LINAC, all with little or no side effects. Immediately after Cyberknife® treatment, almost all patients can go back to work or resume their normal activities.

Like LINAC, Cyberknife® was used as a minimally invasive modality for treating pituitary adenomas. Ji Sun Jan et al. presented in SRT/SBRT meeting held by the radiosurgery society, 27 patients with pituitary adenomas were treated by Cyberknife® and followed for more than a year [37]. Most of them (22 from 27) had undergone a tumor removal operation either by transsphenoidal or transcranial approach. All patients were analyzed using the change in tumor volume, visual acuity, hormonal function, and complications by LINAC. The therapeutic response, as measured by the size of the tumor, was classified as follows, according to guidelines proposed by the Committee of the Brain Tumor

Registry of Japan: complete response (CR: Gd-enhanced area disappears, and no regrowth is recognized at least four weeks after treatment), partial response (PR: Gd-enhanced area is reduced by more than 50%, and maintains this state at least four weeks after treatment), minor response (MR: Gd-enhanced area is reduced from to 25% to 50%, and maintains this state at least four weeks after treatment), no change (NC: less than 50% reduction or less than 25% growth of Gd-enhanced area, maintained at least four weeks after treatment), and progressive disease (PD: more than 35% of Gd-enhanced area). The tumor control rates were calculated by CR + PR + MR + NC/CR + PR + MR + NC + PD. Statistical data from this study revealed that the tumor control rate was 92.3% and Cyberknife® is effective and safe against pituitary adenomas.

Another study confirmed the efficacy of this sophisticated tool was reported by Hiromitsu Iwata et al. They evaluate the clinical outcome of hypofractionated stereotactic radiotherapy (SRT) with Cyberknife® for nonfunctioning pituitary adenoma [38]. After 10 years of Cyberknife® treatment, 100 patients with nonfunctioning pituitary adenoma were treated with hypofractionated SRT. The patient's ages ranged from 16 to 82 years (median, 59 years). Five patients were medically inoperable, and 1 refused surgery; the remaining 94 were recurrent cases or those receiving postoperative adjuvant SRT. Tumor volume ranged from 0.7 to 643 mL (median, 5.1mL). The marginal doses were 17.0 to 21.0 Gy for the 3-fraction schedule and 22.0 to 25.0 Gy for the 5-fraction schedule. The 3-year overall survival and local control rates were 98% and 98% respectively. A post-SRT grade 2 visual disorder occurred in 1 patient. Symptomatic post-SRT hypopituitarism was observed in 3 of 74 patients who had not received hormonal replacement therapy after surgery. From their study, hypofractionated SRT using Cyberknife® appears useful for protecting the visual nerve and neuroendocrine function, especially for tumors located near the optic pathways and large volume adenomas.

Regarding the efficacy between a single dose stereotactic radiosurgery (SRS) like Gamma knife® and multiple doses of fractionated stereotactic radiotherapy (FSRT) like Cyberknife®, both SRS and FSRT represent effective treatment modalities of irradiation for patients with persistent active GH/IGF-I hyper-secretion after surgery and/or during medical therapy, providing comparable high rates of tumor control and endocrinological remission with low morbidity. SRS is a convenient approach for patients with relatively small residual GH-secreting tumors, while FSRT is usually reserved for patients with larger tumors not amenable to SRS [39].

	Gamma Knife®	**CyberKnife®**
	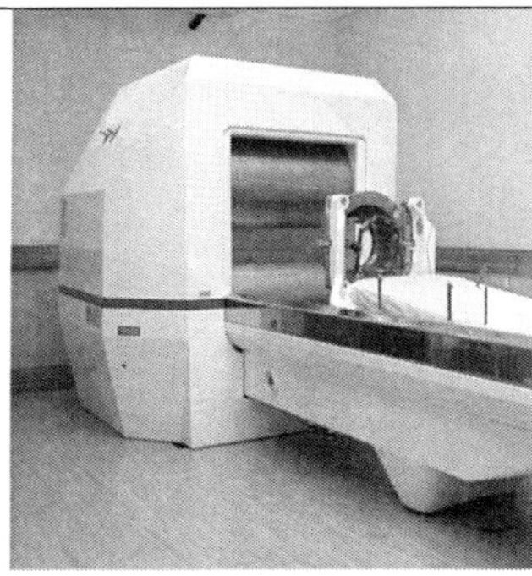	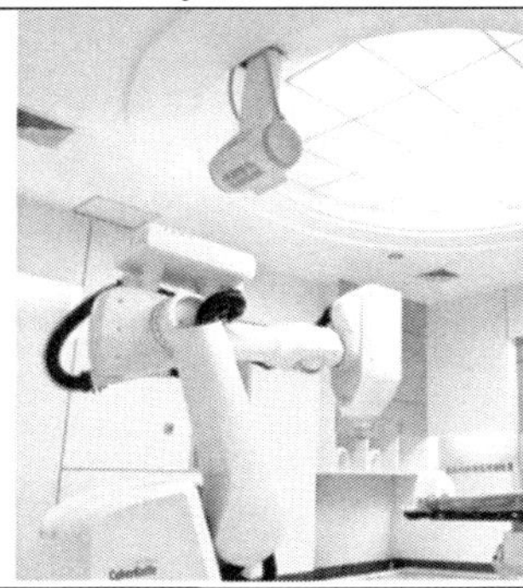
Area coverage	Brain.	Whole body.
Accuracy	The most accurate radiosurgery (SRS). 0.15-0.3 mm. Lowest dose for brain SRS.	High accuracy but not much as compare with Gamma Knife®. mm. Dose *outside* the target area is higher than with Gamma Knife®.
Frame/Frameless	Stereotactic frame is attached to the head to hold it in place for maximum accuracy.	No need for a patient to be still, so no head frame is needed. However to reduce head movement, a custom mask (thermoplastic face mask) that is fixed and shrink-wrapped to the table.
Automatic real-time adjustable software	No real-time software.	Motion management method / Tumor tracking. (Automatically adjusts to the movement by real-time software).
Target position	Confirmed 10 times per second.	Confirmed once every 10 seconds.
Treatment delivered	Only one session.	Single or multiple sessions, over a period of days to weeks. (Fractionated schedule)

	Gamma Knife®	**CyberKnife®**
MR and CT correlation	Exactly: from planning to treatment delivery in 3D since the position is guided by rigid head-frame based.	Relatively: inherently less accurate than Gamma Knife® since the positioning is optically guided. (Dose painting)
Size of lesion	Only small lesion. (Usually < 3 cm.)	Larger lesion available by fractionated schedule.
Planning	Simple.	Complex.
Source	201 Cobalt source. (Radiation)	Single source linear accelerator with robotic arm (6MV LA). (Electricity)
Electricity	Need less electricity.	Need high electricity.

Chapter VII

Role of Radiosurgery in Pituitary Adenoma

Surgical resection or medication is typically the primary treatment modality for pituitary adenomas, especially when the patients have compressive symptoms from mass effect resulting from the adenomas. Surgery is the most proper treatment for non-functioning pituitary adenomas or some functioning pituitary adenomas causing Cushing's disease or acromegaly. In the case of functioning pituitary adenomas, especially prolactinoma, medication may be the treatment of choice for many patients. If functioning pituitary adenomas are not responding to any medication, surgery will be the next option in order to normalize abnormal hormonal levels and alleviate the mass effect of the adenoma. Under modern microscopic or endoscopic technique, neurosurgeons can completely remove the adenoma. For residual or recurrent adenomas, radiosurgery is the next available option. The most common residual adenomas are due to tumor invasion into the surrounding structures that are impossible to resect without significant neurological deficit. Cavernous sinus invasion seems to be the most common surrounding structures that are difficult to remove completely. However, radiosurgery has a prolonged latency, up to years, for its effects and is associated with many sequelae as optic apparatus injury and pituitary gland/stalk injury. But as compared with repeated surgery, radiosurgery may have better outcome.

Remember that a pituitary adenoma is a benign condition and in most cases, surgery is an acceptable method. Use of radiotherapy may cause harm to normal pituitary cells. Judicious use of radiotherapy on a pituitary adenoma is mandatory. Considered role of radiosurgery for a pituitary adenoma in some selected cases:

(1) Intraoperative complete removal but 2 months postoperative MRI assessment confirmed unequivocal complete excision.
(2) For large residual tumor (> 2-3 cm) as postoperative adjuvant.
(3) For small residual tumor (< 2cm), could wait for regular MRI check-up.
(4) Recurrent adenomas
(5) Tumor very close to optic apparatus (<4 mm): Fractionated SRT is suggested.
(6) Inoperable patient (high medical risk for general anesthesia)
(7) Invasive extension (cavernous sinus, para- or suprasellar involvement)
(8) Rejected operation
(9) Functioning adenomas uncontrolled/nonresponsive by medication

The study by Laws ER et al. revealed that radiosurgery offers a tumor growth control rate of approximately 90%, while the reported rates of hormonal normalization for functioning adenomas vary substantially and may be from the widespread differences in endocrinological criteria utilized for post-radiosurgical assessment [40]. As compared with fractionated radiation therapy, stereotactic radiosurgery has lower risks of radiation induced neoplasia and cerebral vasculopathy. And the incidence of other serious complications following radiosurgery is quite low. This supports that radiosurgery may be the best initial treatment in some pituitary adenoma cases.

Summarized by Frederic Castinetti, gamma knife radiosurgery is an effective and safe technique for treating pituitary adenomas [41]. It has a reasonably good anti-secretory and a high antitumoral efficacy, making it a valuable treatment in case of contra-indication or partial efficacy of transsphenoidal surgery. However, they stressed that stereotactic radiosurgery should be reserved only for small lesions, well defined on imaging technique, because its mechanism of action is based on a precise single high dose fraction. When compared to fractionated radiosurgery, the main advantages of stereotactic radiosurgery are the relative rapidity of the effects (with a shorter time to remission) and a theoretically lower risk of adverse effects. However, as indications of both techniques are different, stereotactic radiosurgery and fractionated radiotherapy should not be considered as mutually exclusive, but more as complementary ways to treat different kinds of pituitary adenomas.

Even though stereotactic radiosurgery has many advantages, the drawbacks persist. Delay to remission is still the main drawback and this has to be taken into account at the time of disease management decision. The mean time to remission after radiosurgery is usually about 30-50 months in patients with acromegaly, and 15-30 months in patients with Cushing's disease and prolactinoma. This delay to remission implies that it should be used in patients with low secreting tumors, or in patients for whom an anti-secretory drug is at least partially effective. So, stereotactic radiosurgery should be reserved to tumors with a relatively low level of hypersecretion [42].

According to the "International Radiosurgery Association" guideline in treating pituitary adenomas with stereotactic radiosurgery, patients with pituitary adenomas should be handled with a multidisciplinary team approach with multimodal treatment. Transsphenoidal tumor resection remains the primary recommendation for macroadenomas compressing the optic apparatus or when a rapid reduction in excessive hormone level is required. However about 30% of patients require adjuvant treatment. Fractionated radiation therapy is no longer the best option because it has a prolonged latency (maybe up to 10 years) for its effects, and is associated with many iatrogenic complications: hypopituitarism, visual damage, cerebral vasculopathy, radiation necrosis, potential cognitive effects, and radiation induced tumors. Single session radiosurgery provides better outcome especially in terms of growth control and long-term endocrine control. The latency of the radiation response after radiosurgery is substantially shorter than that of fractionated radiotherapy. This short latency can be managed by adjuvant medication. The risk of hypopituitarism is significantly lower with single session radiosurgery as compared to fractionated radiation therapy. Stereotactic radiosurgery better limits radiation exposure of the surrounding normal brain. In cases of pituitary adenomas near the optic nerves, tracts, or chiasm, Cyberknife® is an excellent tool because of its high precision. Gamma Knife® is typically used for pituitary adenomas located greater than 3-5 mm from these structures.

Even though radiosurgery is considered a minimally invasive treatment for pituitary adenomas, it should be reserved as an additional option when medical or surgical treatments have been exhausted. When patients require radiosurgery, they should be advised about the possible need of endocrinological surveillance and hormonal supplementation for life. And because the response after radiosurgery is extremely slow, they should be closely followed by OPD visits and regular imaging examination.

Chapter VIII

Future Trend of Minimally Invasive Pituitary Surgery (MIPS)

The great leap in neurosurgical operations should be credited to the introduction of the "Hi-end" microscope into the field of neurosurgery. This evolution of the operating microscope began in the late 16th century and by the early 20th century, otolaryngologists became the first surgeons to use the microscope in real clinical surgery. For neurosurgeons, neurosurgical operations were transformed from revolutionary and unorthodox "equipment" into the standard of care of modern neurosurgery [43]. Nowadays, these sophisticated operating microscopes are necessary equipment in many minimally invasive neurosurgical operations.

The next leap in neurosurgical operations was continued by the introduction of the endoscope into the neurosurgical operating theatre. In the beginning of the neuroendoscopic era, it was used in the treatment of hydrocephalus (third ventriculostomy) and intraventricular tumors or cysts. In many cases, the endoscopes were used as an adjunct to operating microscopes for avoiding the blind spot occurring in microscopic neurosurgery. When the neurosurgeons gained more experience with the endoscopic usage, the advantages the endoscopes are self-evident. New designs of the neuroendoscopes and related-instruments have been improved, especially the use of the endoscope as an assisted tool to see around the corners for the main tool for the surgery. Nowadays, neuroendoscopy is widely accepted as standard treatment in many different neurological diseases.

Both the microscopic and endoscopic technique in handling pituitary adenomas are accepted as minimally invasive procedures because surgeons can make smaller incisions or no incision at all to access the surgical site and can be more precise with affiliated equipment, such as fluoroscopes or neuronavigators. Patients get many benefits from minimally invasive procedures such as shorter hospital stay, earlier discharge, quicker recovery periods, minimizing trauma, less blood loss, better cosmetic, and smaller or non-visible incisions that result in less pain and less scarring.

The future surgical trend is to expand the variety of minimally invasive approaches by helping scientists innovate new surgical equipment. One of the most interesting trends is robotic-assisted surgery. The meaning of robotic surgery started with computer-assisted surgery, for example the neuronavigator. When more advanced technologies were applied to the medical field then the robotically-assisted surgery was developed to overcome the limited capabilities of humans in performing very delicate surgery. The most renowned robotic-assisted surgery seemed to be credited to the "da Vinci" surgical system (Figure 35). Sometimes we call it "telesurgery" because the surgery is performed by a surgeon at a remote station, and the surgical tasks are directly performed by a robotic system controlled by the surgeon at the remote station. At the remote station, the surgeon views and controls the main console while the surgical arm unit at the operating bed performs the surgery under the surgeon's control. The da Vinci system is widely used in many abdominal surgical procedures such as prostate surgery, uterine surgery (hysterectomy), thoracic surgery, and cardiothoracic surgery.

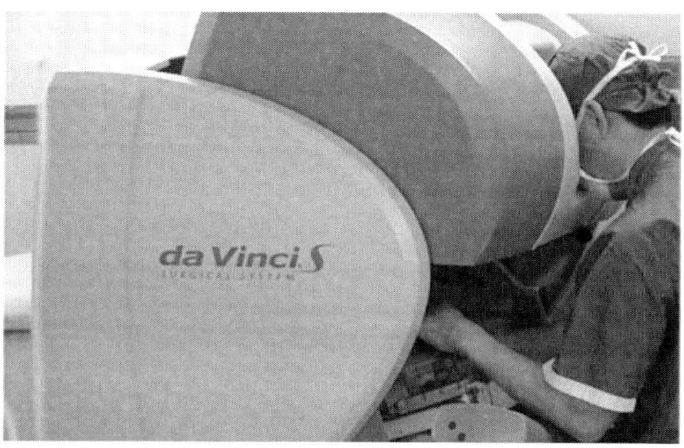

Figure 35. da Vinci surgical system.

From da Vinci comes the "Zeus" robotic surgical system. The system is made up of an ergonomic surgical control console with 3 table-mounted robotic arms. Surgeons control the surgical control console by voice control and touch screen interfaces with 2 monitors. These systems enable surgeons to have greater ability to perform complex and delicate surgical procedures. This system can perform surgical tasks and provide visualization during the endoscopic surgery.

The most recently developed robotic system is the "AESOP" robotic surgical system, and it is the smallest robotic surgical system. Its name stands for "Automated Endoscopic System for Optical Position" hence it is specially designed to work with the endoscopic system and was approved as the first robotic system by the Food and Drug Administration (FDA) to work as an assisted surgeon in the operating theatre.

In the meantime, many institutions around the world are using these sophisticated robotic systems to assist in many surgical procedures. They have great potential to improve the safety and effectiveness of surgeries and lessen the chance of iatrogenic trauma occurring from the limitation of human abilities, especially when working with small and delicate organs or structures. The advantages of the robotic systems are precision enhancement, high accuracy and reliability, fatigueless, more minimally invasive with less pain, less blood loss, less trauma, less anesthesia required, less scarring, less infection rate, and faster recovery period. However, the disadvantage is their price. The cost is very high and very expensive for patients. But in certain operations, they have already proven to be of great value, particularly for very delicate organs. But these technologies are still in their infancy. Their cost effectiveness will improve. The surgical robots can aid surgeons in many ways especially remote surgery, minimally invasive surgery, and unmanned surgery.

For neurosurgical operations, the first robotic surgical system that was used in brain surgery was PUMA 560 as a tool for brain biopsy under CT guidance. The machine still required a surgeon to control the base system by inputting the instructions. The possibility of the applications of robotic systems in neurosurgical operations has been expanded to achieve minimally invasive neurosurgery. For pituitary adenoma surgery, no one denies that the endoscopic transsphenoidal approach using the endoscope and human capability are major keys of success in achieving the best result under a minimally invasive concept. Obviously, every coin has two sides; the endoscopic transsphenoidal approach is associated with flaws and limitations. Two main disadvantages are the lack of 3D vision and the loss of bimanual manipulation. To compensate for 3D vision, a new 3D endoscope is being developed. Regarding loss of bimanual manipulation, the neurosurgeon needs assistance to handle the endoscope during the entire operation but it is still not the best solution because it demands an experienced surgeon to achieve the best result. To alleviate these two limitations, the state-of-art robotic system may be the answer.

As reported by Dallan et al., they applied the da Vinci system in an endoscopic transsphenoidal approach [44]. The bony work is done by traditional endoscopic techniques, given the actual absence of dedicated "robotic" instruments for bone. At this point, the dura of the middle and posterior cranial fossa is exposed and, once opened, a delicate dissection of these areas is performed. As a whole, during dissection, conflict between instruments is minimal. They had concluded that current robotic systems undoubtedly offer the surgeon an excellent view of the surgical field and an incredibly precise and intuitive maneuverability of the arms. The ability to perform precise, tremor-free, bimanual surgery in confined cavities with instrumentation, which exceeds the capabilities of the human hand are the major advantages of the robotic system. But they also pointed out that the cost remains an impediment to the establishment of robotic programs. These costs include purchase, annual maintenance, and cost per case. However, these limitations may be overcome by expanding patient access, increasing the treated numbers. And one day in the future, the operating room will be a place for the patient and robotic system without any doctor inside.

There were many preliminarily reports using robotic-assisted technology for pituitary adenoma surgery. The most recent one is by Raul Wirz et al., their laboratory has developed concentric tube robots for skull base surgery [45]. These consist of concentric prebent nitinol tubes with various end effectors that can be precisely controlled by the operator using a hand held haptic device. In this work, the robot was used to resect a phantom pituitary tumor at a remote location (surgeon in Nashville, Tennessee, United States, robot in Chapel Hill, North Carolina, United States) using an Internet-based data link. Their study demonstrates that a teleoperation with the concentric tube platform, used in a phantom pituitary surgery, was performed at both locations without difficulty. The Internet video stream and robot command instructions were transmitted with sufficient speed and quality. The fact that the robot was 800km away was essentially imperceptible to the surgeon operator. Because of this, an experienced pituitary surgeon was able to perform the resection task without difficulty. Quantitatively, the average latency for the local procedure was 1.1ms with an IAT of 10ms. For the remote procedure, these numbers were 10 and 10.17ms, respectively. The latency for Skype communication was 20ms. Their experiment urged many researchers to develop new technology in aiding neurosurgeons to perform the teleoperation with relative ease in the near future.

From teleoperation to robotic surgical experiment in a cadaveric study, S. Chalongwongse and J. Suthakorn have designed and developed an assisting robot for the endonasal transsphenoidal surgery (ETSS) [46]. Their study is separated into 2 parts: the first is ETSS-workspace analysis, and the second is robot design and implementation for surgical assisting. For ETSS-workspace, an optical tracking system is used to detect motion of surgical instruments while ETSS-procedure is performed in a cadaveric case. Then the workspace and range of motion of instruments are analyzed. Precision and accuracy of their robot are evaluated by an ETSS-phantom that knows the position, orientation of a pituitary tumor and the ETSS-pathway. Their system can also be applied with medical imaging: CT-scan and MRI to analyze optimal pathway of medical tools. The overall results showed that their prototyped robot has the correct range of motion and a small error of the robot's workspace, however improvement is expected with the control system in future work.

Another cadaveric study using robotic assistance in pituitary adenoma surgery was presented in the 2012 Combined Sections Meeting by Randall A. Bly et al., organized by The Triological Society [47]. They created a computer model for cadaver specimens to evaluate the surgical approach by robot. The computer model computed angles between potential transorbital and transnasal portals. The da Vinci robot was used on a dry cadaver skull to perform surgical tasks using transorbital portals. The angles in the robotic arms and different configurations of the tools and endoscope were tested. The Raven II robot was applied to cadaver head specimens to perform a transorbital pituitary resection. They found that transorbital robotic assisted skull base surgery is feasible, as tested with pituitary resections in cadavers. However, future studies are encouraged to improve surgical instrument design and to modify the system to allow access to lesions.

Not only neurosurgeons, but also otolaryngologists tried to operate on the skull base using robotic endoscopic surgery. Ehab Y. Hanna et al. believed that robotic surgery would play an important role for skull base approach [48]. Robotic surgery will allow 2-handed, tremor-free, endoscopic dissection and precise suturing of the dural defect. They operated on 4 human fresh-frozen cadaver specimens. The da Vinci surgical robot was used to place the robotic port and the camera port through one nostril and the other arm ports are placed through the respective anterior and then middle antrostomies (transanstral access). The surgeon performed endoscopic resection under 3-D visualization of the surgical field at the da Vinci's console. The dural defect was also repaired with a meticulous suture technique by the da Vinci robot. The result of their study was excellent. The skull base can be surgically accessed via the robot while the surgeon sits comfortably with good arm support at the console. The 3-D visualization obtained by the dual-channel endoscope at the surgeon's console provided excellent depth perception. They also found that the most significant advantage of this robotic surgery was the ability of the surgeon to perform 2-handed tremor-free endoscopic closure of dural defects. Using robotic platforms in endoscopic surgery has several advantages over standard (manual) endoscopic techniques. Current endoscopic techniques have several ergonomic limitations. Bimanual surgery is only feasible if the endoscope is held by an assistant or a mechanical holder. However, a surgical assistant is preferred because of the constant need to adjust the position (depth and angle) of the endoscope during the surgery. An assistant should have some surgical experience in order to follow the primary surgeon in every step of the operation. Both surgeons have to work within the confined space provided by the nostrils, which in some cases limits ergonomic freedom. Precision during the long period of operation will be limited by fine tremors, especially when using fine instrumentation for delicate dissection of critical neurovascular structures. They concluded that those robotic advantages might expand the indications of minimally invasive endoscopic approaches to the skull base. But future development and refinement of endonasal robotic instrumentation is critical before applying these techniques in the clinical setting.

From all reviewed literature, evolution in robotic surgery demands cutting-edge technology and close contact between doctors and scientists in making surgical robotic platforms. Though robotic assisted surgery is still in development, autonomic or artificial intelligent platforms, which can operate on their own, will surely emerge into the operative theatre. The clear example is supported by the report of Moustris GP et al., their team is going to develop autonomous control of surgical robotic platforms that will offer enhancements such as higher precision, intelligent maneuvers, tissue damage avoidance, etc. [49]. Even though their autonomous robotic systems in surgery are largely at the experimental stage such as miniaturization of robotic arms, proprioception and haptic feedback, new methods for tissue approximation and hemostasis, flexile shafts of robotic instruments, implementation of the natural orifice transluminal endoscopic surgery (NOTES) concept, integration of navigation systems through augmented-reality applications and, finally, autonomous robotic actuation. In their review of literature, we can classify surgical robots into two broad categories, surgical computer-aided design/manufacturing (CAD/CAM) systems, and surgical assistants. Surgical CAD/DCAM systems are designed to assist in planning and intraoperative navigation through reconstruction of preoperative images and formation of three-dimensional (3D) models, registration of the data to the patient in the operative room, and use of robots and image overlay displays to assist in the accurate execution of the planned interventions. Whereas surgical assistant systems can be divided into two classes: surgical extenders, which are operated directly by the surgeon and essentially extend human capabilities in carrying out a variety of surgical tasks, with emphasis on intraoperative decision support and skill enhancement; and auxiliary surgical supports, which work side-by-side with the surgeon and provide support functions such as holding an endoscope.

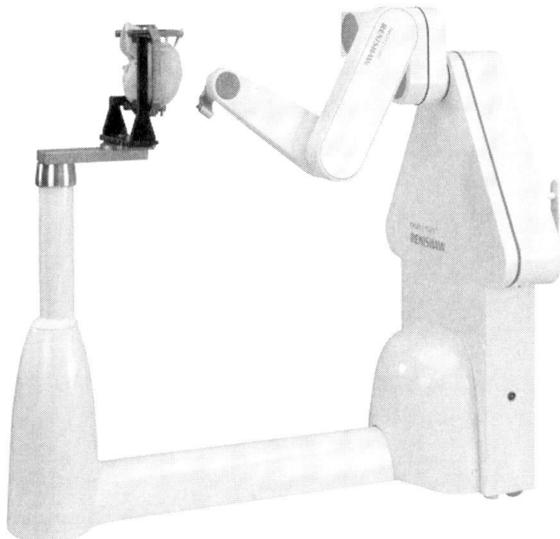

Figure 36. Neuromate®.

According to their study, a division according to autonomous function can be classified into four categories for medical robots, passive robots, semi-active robots, active robots, and remote manipulators. The passive, semi-active, and active robots fall under the surgical CAD/CAM and auxiliary surgical support categories, while the remote manipulators are classified as the surgical extender. The passive robots provide only support action for surgeons; they cannot perform any autonomous or active actions. But semi-active robots are closely related to the assistant surgeons that can provide some tasks such as holding a tool or equipment during the operation. Active robots can perform an autonomous task on their own without direct interaction with the surgeon. Cyberknife® is the best example for this type of robot. However, the active robots are still limited whereas the most common surgical robots that were used in the operating theatres nowadays are remote manipulators or surgical extenders. The da Vinci® system is the most well-known commercial robot of this type. With the da Vinci®, a surgeon controls the slave robot at the master console far from the patient bed, the slave will move its arms after the controlled commanded. The surgeon views the operative field via the endoscope that is usually high-definition 3D images. With this maneuver, the robot will compensate fine movements that ordinary human cannot do.

From the neurosurgical perspective, computers played an important role for many years. The most outstanding system is image-guided technology, which has been used as an adjunct for many neurosurgical operations. The neuronavigator is the best example. With this technology, the surgical instruments were guided in real time by the relationship between the frame and lesion observed in the image. From frame to frameless, frameless image-guided technology uses invisible optical trackers for real time navigation without the use of any fiducial markers. This intraoperative real time navigation creates much less invasive neurosurgical operations with high accuracy reliability.

Other than image-guided technology, sophisticated robot technology was created to aid neurosurgeons in the functional neurosurgical procedure. The Neuromate® stereotactic robot is the mentioned platform (Figure 36). It has been used especially in electrode implantation procedures for deep brain stimulation (DBS) and stereoelectroencephalography (SEEG) as well as stereotactic applications in neuroendoscopy, biopsy, radiosurgery, transcranial magnetic stimulation (TMS), and many other functional neurosurgical procedures. The Neuromate® is capable of delivering greater accuracy and consistency than other conventional methods, improving outcomes and minimizing patients' trauma. It supports both frame-based and frameless modes of stereotactic surgery. Both general and local anesthesia is compatible with the Neuromate®. The difficult operations that required consistent, rapid, and precise targeting can be accomplished by the Neuromate® with ease. Moreover, the Neuromate® is supplied with a navigation system that supports both 2D and 3D systems. It was the first neurobotic device to be approved by FDA, as well as the first to be commercially available. Its platform consists of:

- Robotic arm
- Robotic base
- Central control unit for the arm
- Visualized workstation
- Software for planning and position simulation
- Ultrasound system
- Specific localizers
- Head frame + base

However, the main drawback of Neuromate® is the same as other robotic devices. The cost-to-benefit ratio is a huge problem in using robotic devices. It is too expensive for the hospital to invest in for their rather simple tasks with poor-decision-making capabilities of the robot. The current poor human-to-machine interface and high cost-to-benefit ratio has ultimately limited the integration of robots into routine neurosurgical practice.

Chapter IX

Future Robotic Endoscopic Surgery

Since a novel 3-D visualization system for endoscopic endonasal transsphenoidal surgery was already launched into commercial surgical market, it had significant advantages over traditional 2D endoscopic surgery including better realistic vision, depth perception, and high precision. A combination of 3D endoscopes and robotic systems would be the best answer for high precision surgical procedures. Robotic systems have the capacity to both assist and perform endoscopic nasal surgery via a master-slave interface. Robotic master-slave systems offer advantages of high dexterity and precision, tremor elimination, combined with an excellent field of view afforded by endoscopes [50]. The da Vinci surgical system should be the best example in proving the benefit of this combination. However, the da Vinci surgical system still has some drawbacks for neuroendoscopic surgery, particularly its size and difficulty in instrument exchange. The latest attempt in improving the robotic endoscopic surgery is the innovation of prototype robots with the capacity to handle the endoscope autonomously via speech command from the surgeon, freeing the surgeon to operate bimanually with traditional instruments. The active bending endoscope robot systems circumvent the limitation of the single pivot point at the nostril by offering angles of view up to 180 degrees on the same endoscope. Definitely, the robotic endoscopic surgery will be promising for minimally invasive neuro-surgery.

Pros and Cons of Robotic Surgery

Since robotic surgery is fairly new, and most of them are in clinical research, only some hospitals and institutions can afford it. Moreover, many obstacles and disadvantages must be resolved before their clinical use is undoubtedly proven. To the best of the present knowledge, the pros and cons of robotic surgery can be summarized as detailed.

Pros of Robotic Surgery

(1) Painless, pain-free, minimal pain surgery
(2) Fast recovery
(3) Short hospital stays
(4) High precision and safety: human hands have tremors but robot arms don't shake.
(5) Less infection rate due to small opening (incision)
(6) Less or minimal blood loss
(7) Better cosmetic, less scarring
(8) Step over unmanned surgery because of the efficacy of robot.
(9) Convenience: robotic platforms enable surgeons to have better control over surgical equipment and also enable them to be less tired in difficult operations.

Cons of Robotic Surgery

(1) High cost: this seems to be the main drawback of robotic surgery but when it is widely used, the cost will be lowered.
(2) Special skill is required. Since robotic surgery is based on sophisticated technology, surgeons demand extra-training to control the robot.
(3) Some operations will consume a lot of time then compared to the operation performed by ordinary surgeons.
(4) For telesurgery, the main console should be in close contact with the robotic unit (arm) as much as possible to reduce the time lapse between the instructions given from the console to the arm.
(5) Size does matter: the overall sizes of robotic units are still the big problem. They still need much improvement to overcome this

disadvantage. Someday in the near future, well-established robotic units will be launched into the commercial market.

(6) "Not" user friendly: Most robotic platforms used in many institutions are not user friendly. Their sizes are huge, and the platforms are very complicated. Despite the potential of robotic surgery, so much expertise is required; hence these robots have not yet been widely accepted. Scientists must overcome this problem by innovating user-friendly platforms that facilitate the surgical procedures.

However, when enough improvement becomes reality and the advantages clearly outweigh the disadvantages, robotic surgery will be firmly established as one of the standard surgical procedures for the sake of mankind. Definitely, in the near future, robotic assisted or pure robotic surgery will play an important role, not even for pituitary adenomas surgery, but for many scopes of neurosurgical operation. It allows precise, accurate, and repeated motions with decreased fatigue of surgeons. High accuracy, delicate and fine movement, and more flexibility make it more reasonable for critical organ surgery like the central nervous system, especially the brain. Presently, intensive research is underway all over the world. Better image-guidance, sophisticated computer technology, close collaboration between physicist, biologist, scientist, and medical personnel will allow greater compatibility in neurosurgical operation. The robotic technology will handle a larger scale of surgery than previously limited by the natural dexterity of human capability. The newly developed machines are going to launch into the market and be ready to treat the untreatable disease. These machines may look like the fantastic equipment we saw in Hollywood movies. It can perform the tasks that seem to be impossible when being done by human surgeons. With improvements in computer technology, engineering, medical knowledge, along with the collaboration of neurosurgeons worldwide, the age of digital robotic neurosurgery is certain to come sooner or later.

References

[1] Hung Tzu Wen, Evandro de Oliveira, Helder Tedeschi, Francisco C. Andrade Jr., Albert L. Rhoton Jr., (2001). The pterional approach: Surgical anatomy, operative technique, and rationale. *Operative Techniques in Neurosurgery* 4(2), 60-72.

[2] P. Grunert., (2013). Review Article: From the Idea to Its Realization: The Evolution of Minimally Invasive Techniques in Neurosurgery. *Minimally Invasive Surgery* Volume 2013 (2013), Article ID 171369, 18 pages. http://dx.doi.org/10.1155/2013/171369.

[3] Peris-Celda M., Kucukyuruk B., Monroy-Sosa A., Funaki T., Valentine R., Rhoton AL Jr., (2013). The Recesses of the Sellar Wall of the Sphenoid Sinus and Their Intracranial Relationships. *Neurosurgery* 73 [ONS Suppl 2]:ons117-ons131. doi:10.1227//NEU.0000000000000184.

[4] Ozcan T., Yilmazlar S., Aker S, Korfali E., (2010). Surgical limits in transnasal approach to opticocarotid region and planum sphenoidale: an anatomic cadaveric study. *World Neurosurg.* 73(4):326-33. doi:10.1016/j.wneu.2010.01.015.

[5] Esposito F., Dusick JR., Fatemi N., Kelly DF., (2007). Graded repair of cranial base defects and cerebrospinal fluid leaks in transsphenoidal surgery. *Neurosurgery* 60(4 Suppl 2):295-303; discussion 303-4.

[6] Gondim JA., Almeida JP., Albuquerque LA., Schops M., Gomes E., Ferraz T., Sobreira W., Kretzmann MT., (2011). Endoscopic endonasal approach for pituitary adenoma: surgical complications in 301 patients. *Pituitary* 14(2):174-83. doi:10.1007/s11102-010-0280-1.

[7] Blake Charles Walker, Mark Hornyak, David S. Hong, Matthew Schreckinger, Murali Guthikonda, Sandeep Mittal, Nicholas J. Szerlip.,

Risks of Diabetes Insipidus Following Endoscopic Transsphenoidal Surgery. Retrieved from http://w3.cns.org/dp/2012CNS/1222.pdf

[8] Shah S., Har-El G., (2001). Diabetes insipidus after pituitary surgery: incidence after traditional versus endoscopic transsphenoidal approaches. *Am J Rhinol.* 15(6):377-9.

[9] Cappabianca P., Cavallo LM., de Divitiis E., (2004). Endoscopic endonasal transsphenoidal surgery. *Neurosurgery* 55:933-40.

[10] Arbolay OL., Rojas Manresa JL., Galvez YH., (2013). Endonasal endoscopic approach in pituitary adenomas: surgical results. *Neurosci Discov* 1:5. doi:http://dx.doi.org/10.7243/2052-6946-1-5.

[11] Joseph B. Eby, Sung Tae Cha., Fully endoscopic transnasal-transsphenoidal pituitary stalk surgery. Retrieved from http://www.skullbaseinstitute.com/papers/fully-endoscopic-transnasal-transsphenoidal.htm.

[12] Yang Gao, Chunlong Zhong, Yu Wang, Siyi Xu, Yang Guo, Chenyang Dai, Yan Zheng, Yong Wang, Qizhong zLuo, Jiyao Jiang., (2014). Endoscopic versus microscopic transsphenoidal pituitary adenoma surgery: A meta-analysis. *World J Surg Oncol.* 12:94. doi:10.1186/1477-7819-12-94.

[13] Heroes RC., (2011). The supraorbital "keyhole" approach. *J Neurosurg.* 114: 850-851.

[14] Ryan Ormond, Costas G. Hadjipanayis., (2013). The Supraorbital Keyhole Craniotomy through an Eyebrow Incision: Its Origins and Evolution. Minimally Invasive Surgery. Article ID 296469, 11 pages. Retrieved from http://www.hindawi.com/journals/mis/2013/296469/#B36

[15] Wiedemayer H., Sandalcioglu IE., Wiedemayer H., Stolke D., (2004). The supraorbital keyhole approach via an eyebrow incision for resection of tumors around the sella and the anterior skull base. *Minim Invasive Neurosurg* 47: 221-5.

[16] Ormond DR., Hadjipanayis CG., (2013). The supraorbital keyhole craniotomy through an eyebrow incision: its origins and evolution. *Minim Invasive Surg* 2013:296469. doi: 10.1155/2013/296469.

[17] Fatemi N., Dusick JR., Paiva Neto MA., Malkasian D., Kelly DF., (2009). Endonasal versus supraorbital keyhole removal of craniopharyngiomas and tuberculum sellae meningiomas. *Neurosurgery* 64: 269-86.

[18] A. Perneczky, (1992). Planning strategies for the suprasellar region: philosophy of approaches. *Neurosurgeon* 11:343–348.

[19] ZHANG Mao-zhi, WANG Lei, ZHANG Wei, QI Wei, WANG Rong, HAN Xiao-di, ZHAO Ji-zong., (2004). The supraorbital keyhole approach with eyebrow incisions for treating lesions in the anterior fossa and sellar region. *Chinese Medical Journal* 117(3): 323-326.

[20] Jouanneau Emmanuel, Messerer Mahmoud, Berhouma Moncef, (2011). Endoscopic Endonasal Skull Base Surgery: Current State of the Art and Future Trends, *Advances in Endoscopic Surgery*, Prof. Cornel Iancu (Ed.), ISBN: 978-953-307-717-8, InTech. Retrieved from: http://www.intechopen.com/books/advances-inendoscopic-surgery/endoscopic-endonasal-skull-base-surgery-current-state-of-the-art-and-future-trends.

[21] Heung Sik Park, Sang Kyu Park, Young Min Han., (2009). Microsurgical Experience with Supraorbital Keyhole Operations on Anterior Circulation Aneurysms. *J Korean Neurosurg Soc* 46:103-108.

[22] Ramos-Zúñiga, Velázquez H., Barajas MA., López R., Sánchez E., Trejo S., (2002). Trans-supraorbital approach to supratentorial aneurysms. *Neurosurgery* 51(1):125-131.

[23] El Shafei H.I., (2011). Anterolateral Mini Fronto-Orbito-Zygomatic Craniotomy via an Eyebrow Incision in Pediatrics: Technical Notes and Evaluation. *Pediatr Neurosurg* 47:248-253.

[24] Wongsirisuwan M., (2011). What is the Better Minimally Invasive Surgery in Pituitary Surgery: Endoscopic Endonasal Transsphenoidal Approach or Keyhole Supraorbital Approach? *J Med Assoc Thai* 94(7): 888-95.

[25] Sazgar AA., Massah J., Sadeghi M., Bagheri A., Rasool E., (2008). The incidence of concha bullosa and the correlation with nasal septal deviation. *B-ENT* 4: 87-91.

[26] Stallman JS., Lobo JN., Som PM., (2004). The incidence of concha bullosa and its relationship to nasal septal deviation and paranasal sinus disease. *Am J Neuroradiol* 25: 1613-8.

[27] van Lindert EJ., Ingels K., Mylanus E., Grotenhuis JA., (2010). Variations of endonasal anatomy: relevance for the endoscopic endonasal transsphenoidal approach. *Acta Neurochir(Wien)* 152:1015-20.

[28] Brian B. Ronson, Reinhard W. Schulte, Khanh P. Han, Lilia N. Loredo, James M. Slater, Jerry D. Slater, (2006). Fractionated proton beam irradiation of pituitary adenomas. *International Journal of Radiation Oncology* 63(2):425-434.

[29] Jason P. Sheehan, Douglas Kondziolka, John Flickinger, L. Dade Lunsford., (2003). Radiosurgery for Nonfunctioning Pituitary Adenoma. *Neurosurg Focus* 14(5). Retrieved from http://www.medscape.com/viewarticle/456136

[30] Raef FA Hafez, Magad S. Morgan, Osama M. Fahmy., (2014). Gamma knife surgery in management of secretory pituitary adenoma preliminary evaluation of role, efficacy and safety. *Neuroscience Discovery* 2(1):4. http://dx.doi.org/10.7243/2052-6946-2-4

[31] Glenn A. Tung, Georg Noren, Jeffrey M. Rogg, Ivor M.D. Jackson, (2001). MR imaging of pituitary adenomas after Gamma Knife stereotactic radiosurgery. *American Journal of Roentgenology* 177: 919-924.

[32] Tatsuya Kobayashi., (2009). Long-term results of stereotactic gamma knife radiosurgery for pituitary adenomas. Specific strategies for different types of adenoma. *Progress in neurological surgery* 02/2009; 22:77-95. DOI: 10.1159/000163384

[33] Runge MJ., Maarouf M., Hunsche S., Kocher M., Ruge MI., El Majdoub F., Treuer H., Mueller RP., Voges J., Sturm V., (2012). LINAC-radiosurgery for nonsecreting pituitary adenomas. Long-term results. *Strahlenther Onkol.* 188(4):319-25.

[34] Muramatsu J., Yoshida M., Shioura H., Kawamura Y., Ito H., Takeuchi H., Kubota T., Maruyama I., (2003). Clinical results of LINAC-based stereotactic radiosurgery for pituitary adenoma. *Nihon Igaku Hoshasen Gakkai Zasshi* 63(5):225-30.

[35] Yoon Sei-Chul, Suh Tae-Suk, Jang Hong-Seok, Dhung Su-Mi, Kim Yeon-Shil, Ryu Mi-Ryeong, choi Kyu-Ho, son Ho-Yong, Kim Moon-chan, Shinn Kyung-Sub., (1998). Clinical results of 24 pituitary macrosdenomas with linac-based stereotactic radiosurgery. *International Journal of Radiation Oncology* 41(4):849-853.

[36] Mathis, S., Eisner, W., (2010). Gamma Knife versus adapted linear accelerators: A comparison of two radiosurgical applications. *HTA-Projektbericht* 4. Retrieved from http://eprints.hta.lbg.ac.at/901/

[37] Ji Sun Jang, Moon Chan Kim, Kyung Jin Lee. *Long term results of pituitary adenomas after Cyberknife treatment.* Presented in SRT/SBRT meeting.

[38] Iwata H., Sato K., Tatewaki K., Yokota N., Inoue M., Baba Y., Shibamoto Y., (2011). Hypofractionated stereotactic radiotherapy with CyberKnife for nonfunctioning pituitary adenoma: high local control with low toxicity. *Neuro-oncol.* 13(8):916-22. doi: 10.1093/neuonc/nor055.

[39] G. Minniti,C. Scaringi, D. Amelio, R. Maurizi Enrici., (2012). Stereotactic Irradiation of GH-Secreting Pituitary Adenomas. *International Journal of Endocrinology.* http://dx.doi.org/10.1155/2012/482861

[40] Laws ER., Sheehan JP., Sheehan JM., Jagnathan J., Jane JA Jr., Oskouian R., (2004). Stereotactic radiosurgery for pituitary adenomas: a review of the literature. *J Neurooncol.* 69(1-3):257-72.

[41] Castinetti F., (2010). Gamma Knife Radiosurgery in Pituitary Adenomas: Why, Who, and How to Treat? Retrieved from http://www.discovery medicine.com/Frederic-Castinetti/2010/08/04/gamma-knife-radiosurgery-in-pituitary-adenomas-why-who-and-how-to-treat/

[42] Castinetti F., Regis J., Dufour H., Brue T., (2010). Role of stereotactic radiosurgery in the management of pituitary adenomas. *Nat Rev Endocrinol* 6(4):214-23.

[43] Kriss TC., Kriss VM., (1998). History of the operating microscope: from magnifying glass to microneurosurgery. *Neurosurgery* 42(4):899-907; discussion 907-8.

[44] I. Dalln, P. Castelnuovo, C. Vicini, M. Tschabitscher., (2011). The natural evolution of endoscopic approaches in skull base surgery: robotic-assisted surgery? *Acta Otorhinolaryngol Ital.* 31(6): 390–394.

[45] Raul Wirz, Luis Torres, Philip Swaney, Hunter Gilbert, Ron Alterovitz, Robert Webster, Kyle Weaver, Paul Russell., (2015). Teleoperation of Concentric Tube Robots for Skull Base Applications: Pituitary Surgery at a Distance? *J Neurol Surg B* 76-A151. doi: 10.1055/s-0035-1546615

[46] S. Chalongwongse, J. Suthakorn., (2014). Workspace determination and robot design of a prototyped surgical robotic system based on a cadaveric study in endonasal transsphenoidal surgery. *International conference on robotics and biometics.* December 5-10, Bali, Indonesia.

[47] Randall A Bly, David Su, Thomas S Lendvay, Diana Friedman, Blake Hannaford, Manuel Ferreira, Kris S Moe., (2012). Transorbital robotic skull base surgery: a preclinical study. *2012 Combined Sections Meeting. The Triological Socitey.* Jan 26-28, 2012. Miami Beach, Florida. Retrieved from http://www.triomeetingposters.org/wp-content/uploads/2012/12/057.pdf

[48] Ehab Y. Hanna, Christopher Holsinger, Franco DeMonte, Michael Kupferman., (2007). Robotic endoscopic surgery of the skull base: A novel surgical approach. *Arch Otolaryngol Head Neck Surg.* 133(12):1209-1214.

[49] Moustris GP., Hiridis SC., Deliparachos KM., Konstantinidis KM., (2011). Evolution of autonomous and semi-autonomous robotic surgical systems: a review of the literature. *Int J Med Robotics Comput Assist Surg.* 7:375-392.

[50] Alexander Yao., (2013). Endoscopic nasal surgery-a surgical fashion or genuine progress? Retrieve from https://entuk.org/sites/default/files/files/ ENT UK essay Alex Yao.pdf.

Index

C

D

E

F

G

H

I

J

K

L

M

N

O

P

R

S

T